Hazardous Waste Operations and Emergency Response

This training manual is designed for students who will or are routine site employee's either maximum or minimal exposure, Non-routine Site employee's and General Site Employees. This book is also designed for all employees working on Hazardous Material Sites, who may be exposed to hazardous substances, health hazards, or safety hazards and their supervisors and management responsible for the site shall receive training meeting the requirements before they are permitted to engage in hazardous waste operation that could expose them to hazardous substances, safety or health hazards, and they shall receive review training as specified in the OSHA 1926 training standards guideline in this book as specified. It includes personnel who are involved with the investigation and the remediation of uncontrolled hazardous waste sites. To lesser extent, it is designed for personnel who respond to accidents or to releases of hazardous materials. It provides basic information needed to meet the requirements of 29CFR1910.120 "Hazardous Waste Operations and Emergency Response".

After completing your level of training, students will be able to:

- **Identify methods and procedures for recognizing, evaluating, and controlling hazardous substances.**
- **Identify concepts, principals and guidelines to properly protect site and response personnel**
- **Discuss regulations and actions levels to ensure the health and safety of the workers**
- **Discuss the fundamentals needed to develop organizational structure and stand operation procedures**
- **Demonstrate the selections and use of dermal and respiratory protection equipment**
- **Demonstrate the use and calibration of direct-reading air monitoring instruments**
- **References to products and manufactures are for illustration purposes only and do not imply endorsement by the Occupational Safety & Health Administration, the US Environmental Protection Agency or your instructors or the training provider.**

Published with permission of OSHA & EPA by:
ehsMaterials.com, Inc.
P.O. Box 447, DuQuoin, IL 62832
Ph: 800/530-1161   Fax: 888/494-6140

HAZWOPER

HAZARD WASTE OPERATIONS & EMERGENCY RESPONSE

Chapter 1 – Hazard Recognition

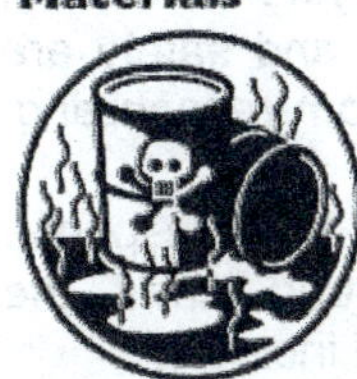

Hazardous Materials

A hazardous material incident is a situation in which a hazardous material is or can escape into the environment. Hundreds of thousands of different chemicals are produced, stored, transported, and used annually. Because of the hazardous nature of many of them, safeguards are established to prevent them from causing harm. If these safeguards are accidentally or purposefully disregarded, the material is no longer under effective control. Then a situation is established that can have dangerous effects. Hazardous material incidents vary considerably. Considerations are chemicals and quantities involved, types of hazard, response efforts required, number of responders needed, and effects produced. They may require immediate control measures (emergency) or long-term cleanup activities (remedial action) to restore acceptable conditions.

Activities that is required when responding to incidents can be divided into five broad, interacting elements.

- **Recognition**: identification of the substance involved and the characteristics which determine its degree of hazard.

- **Evaluation:** impact or risk the substance poses to the workers, public health, and the environment.

- **Control**: methods to eliminate or reduce the impact of the incident.

- **Information**: knowledge gained about the conditions or circumstances particular to an incident. Information is often times called intelligence. In a response, you gather intelligence and disseminate it.

- **Safety**: protection of responders from harm.

These elements make up a system - an orderly arrangement of components that interact to accomplish a task. In response work, the task is to prevent or reduce the impact of the incident on people, property, and the environment, and to restore conditions to as near normal as possible. To achieve this goal, response personnel undertake a variety of activities, for example, firefighting, sampling, developing safety plans, erecting fences, installing a physical treatment system, record keeping, evaluation, etc. These activities are all related; what occurs in one affects or is affected by the others.

Five elements classify all response activities. Recognition, evaluation, and control describe performance-oriented elements. There is an outcome - a sample needs to be collected, a treatment system installed, a chemical identified, or a risk determined. Information and safety are supportive elements. They are the results that come from recognizing, evaluating, and controlling.

Understanding the system provides some insight into how response activities relate to each other. It helps explain, in broad terms, the processes involved in responding to a hazardous material incident.

THE INCIDENT RESPONSE SYSTEM

Recognition

Recognizing the type and degree of the hazard present is usually one of the first steps in responding to an incident. The substance involved must be identified. Then the physical and chemical properties that may make it hazardous – capable of causing harm – are determined. These

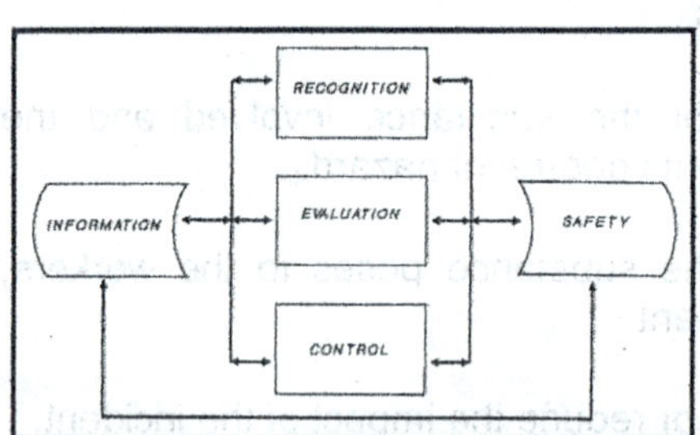

inherent properties are used, on a preliminary basis, to predict the behavior and anticipated problems associated with a material.

Recognition may be easy. For example, the placard on a railroad tank car carrying a hazardous material is used to quickly identify its content. At a hazardous waste site, which may contain hundreds of different chemicals, complete identification is more difficult. The element of recognition, therefore, involves the use of all available information (e.g., sampling results, historical data, visual observation, instruments, package labels, shipping manifests, existing documentation, witnesses, and other sources) to identify the substances.

An incident involves more than the mere presence of a hazardous material. It is a situation in which the normal safeguards associated with the materials are compromised, thus creating the chance of undesirable effects. For instance, gasoline can do harm because its vapors can ignite and explode. However, the usual safety techniques for handling gasoline prevent this from happening. Problems caused by the release of gasoline into the environment can be anticipated based on its chemical and physical properties. The harm that gasoline will do if released at a site, however, depends on site-specific conditions.

Thousands of substances exhibit one or more characteristics of flammability, radioactivity, corrosiveness, toxicity, or other properties that classify them as hazardous. For any particular hazardous category, the degree of hazard varies depending on the substance. The degree of hazard is a relative measure of how hazardous a substance is. For instance, the Immediately Dangerous to Life or Health (IDLH) concentration of butyl acetate in air is 10,000 parts per million (ppm); the IDLH for sulfur dioxide is 100 ppm. Sulfur dioxide, therefore, is much more acutely toxic (has a higher degree of hazard) when inhaled at IDLH concentrations than butyl acetate. Vapors from butyl acetate, however, have a higher degree of explosive hazard those tetrachloroethane vapors, which are not explosive.

Once the substance(s) have been identified, its hazardous properties and its degree of hazard is determined using reference material. Although appropriate references give information about the substance's physical/chemical properties and may give indications of its environmental behavior, additional data is required. Most frequently, monitoring and sampling data are used to: (1) identify substances, (2) determine concentrations, (3) confirm dispersion patterns, and (4) verify the presence of material.

Evaluation

Recognition provides basic data about the substance. Evaluation is defined as determining its effects, or potential impact, on public health, property, and the environment. A hazardous substance is a threat due to its physical and chemical characteristics. Its actual impact, however, depends on the location of the release, on weather, and other site-specific conditions. Two measures of impact are: (1) the adverse effects that have occurred, and (2) the potential impact of the substance if released. Risk is the chance of harm being done, a measure of the potential impact or effect. The presence of a hazardous substance is a risk, but if the material is under control, the risk is low; if uncontrolled, the risk increases. For harm to be done, a critical receptor must be exposed to the uncontrolled material, as when people live in the area, property will be impacted, or a sensitive ecological habitat will be affected. Chlorine gas, for instance, is highly toxic and represents a risk. If chlorine gas is released in a densely populated area. the risk to people is very great, while the human risk associated with a release of chlorine gas in an unpopulated area is very low. If the substance was carbon dioxide rather than chlorine, the human risk in both situations would be substantially less, since carbon dioxide is much less toxic than chlorine.

Evaluating risk in these two examples is relatively simple. Much more complex are those episodes where many compounds are involved and a higher degree of uncertainty exists regarding their behavior in the environment and their contact with and effects on receptors. For instance: what is the risk if a few thousand people drink from a waste supply obtained from an aquifer underlying soil containing a few parts per billion of styrene?

The completeness of information must also be assessed. Is additional sampling and monitoring of air, water, and soil necessary to provide more comprehensive information on what the material is, where it is, how it moves through the environment, what it will contact, and what is the associated risk? To evaluate completely the effects of a hazardous materials incident, all substances must be identified, their dispersion pathways established, and for toxic chemicals, concentrations determined. Risk is then assessed based on exposure (or potential exposure) to the public or other critical receptors.

Identifying the materials involved in an incident and evaluating the impact the incident may have, is frequently termed site characterization. Site characterization may be easy and rapid, or as in the case of an abandoned waste site, a process that may take a long time to completely accomplish.

Control

Control is a method (or methods) that prevents or reduces the impact of the incident. Preliminary control actions are instituted as rapidly as possible in emergency situations. As additional information is developed through recognition and evaluation, initial control actions are modified or others instituted. Releases that do not require immediate action allow more time for planning and instituting remedial measures. Control measures include physical, chemical, and biological treatment and cleanup techniques for restoring the area to prerelease conditions. It also includes public health countermeasures, for example, evacuation or the shutdown of a drinking water supply, to prevent contact of people with the substance.

Information

An integral part of response is information. All response activities evolve having information that is readily available or subsequently obtained. Information is a support element to recognition, evaluation, and control. It is an input to the three performance elements and provides data for decision-making. It is also an outcome of these elements. A sample is collected and analyzed. The results provide an input to determine treatment options, an outcome. Information comes from three sources:

- **Intelligence**: Information obtained from existing records or documentation, placards, labels, signs, special configuration of containers, visual observations, technical reports, and others.

- **Direct-reading instruments**: Information relatively quickly obtained from instruments.

- **Sampling**; Information obtained from collecting representative portions of appropriate media or material and subsequent laboratory analysis.

Information acquisition, analyses, and decision-making are iterative processes that define the extent of the problem and the array of possible response actions. For incident response to be effective, an information base must be established which is accurate, valid, and timely. Throughout the lifetime of the incident, a continuous stream of information is collected, processed, and applied. Sound decisions based upon (1) receipt and evaluation of good information, and (2) development of a good knowledge base concerning the situation.

Safety

All hazardous material responses pose varying dangers to responder. An important consideration in all response activities is to protect the health and safety of the responders. To do this requires that the chemical and physical hazards associated with each operation be assessed and methods implemented to prevent or reduce hard to responders. Safety considerations are an input to every activity that and are an outcome of each response activity. For example, an outcome of identifying a specific chemical may be changes in safety requirements. Each response organization must have an effective health and safety program including medical surveillance and health monitoring, appropriate safety equipment, standardized safety procedures, and an active training program.

Relationship of Elements

Recognition, evaluation, control, information, and safety describe the five elements of response. Each includes a variety of activities or operations. Elements are not necessarily sequential steps for responding. In some situations, control measures can start before the substances are completely identified. In others, a more thorough evaluation of the material's dispersion needs to be completed before effective control actions can be determined. Likewise, safety measures for workers may be instituted before the materials are identified or all the hazardous conditions are fully known.

Each element and activity are interrelated A dike (control), to contain the runoff water from fighting a fire at a warehouse suspected of containing pesticides, is built. Once it is determined that the runoff contains no hazardous chemicals (recognition), or that concentrations in the runoff are below acceptable values (evaluation), no treatment is necessary and the dike is removed. This knowledge (information) also changes the safety requirements for responders (safety).

 A constant flow of information is needed to characterize the incident and to make decisions. For example, an option to use carbon absorption for waste treatment may require additional sample collection and analysis to identify completely the substances involved. In turn, this would require reevaluating the effectiveness of carbon absorption for the identified chemicals.

Additional information regarding where and how the substance is migrating may change the requirements for sampling.

The response system is a concept explaining, in general terms, the processes involved in incident response. All responses require the performance elements of recognizing, evaluating, and controlling. To support these, information is needed and responder safety must be considered.

CHEMICAL HAZARDS

Chemical hazards may be classified according to one of many groups. These groups may include toxic, fire and explosive, corrosive, and chemical reactive. A material may elicit more than one chemical hazard. For example, toxic vapors can be released during chemical fires. The hazard may be a result of the physical/chemical properties of the material or of its chemical reactivity with other materials or the environment to which it is exposed.

Toxic Hazards

Toxic materials cause local or systemic detrimental effects in an organism. Exposure to such materials does not always result in death, although that is often the most immediate concern. Types of toxic hazards are categorized by the physiological effect they have on the organism. A material may induce more than one physiological response that may include: asphyxiation, irritation allergic sensitization, systemic poisoning, mutagenesis, teratogenesis, and carcinogenesis.

The likelihood that any of these effects will be experienced by an organism depends on: (1) the inherent toxicity of the material itself (as measured by its lethal dose); (2) the magnitude of the exposure (acute or chronic); and (3) the route of exposure (ingestion, inhalation, skin absorption).

Fire and Explosion Hazards

Combustibility is the ability of a material to act as a fuel. Materials that can be readily ignited and sustain a fire are considered combustible. Those that do not are called noncombustible. Three components are required for combustion to allow ignition and to maintain the burning process. Combustion is the chemical reaction that requires heat to proceed:

$$heat$$
$$fuel + oxygen \longrightarrow products$$

Heat is supplied either by the ignition source and maintained by the combustion, or is from an external source. The relationship of these three components is illustrated by the fire triangle. Most fires can be extinguished by removing one of the three components. For example, water applied to a fire removes the heat, thereby extinguishing the fire. When a material by itself generates enough heat to self-ignite and combust, spontaneous combustion occurs, either as a fire or an explosion.

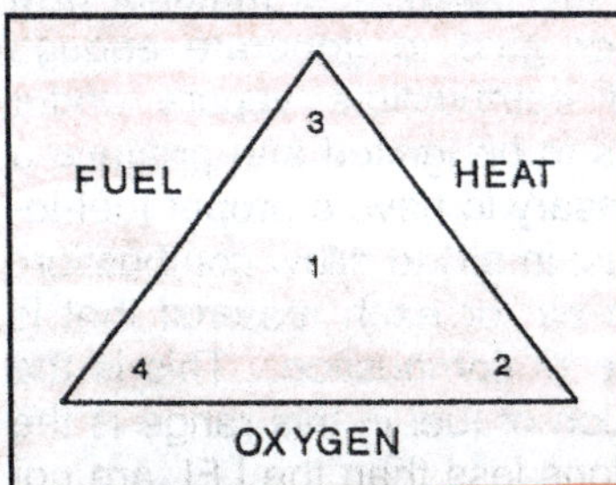

FIRE TRIANGLE

While oxygen is the usual oxidizing agent during the combustion process, there are chemicals that can burn without oxygen being present. For example, calcium, and aluminum will burn in nitrogen. Therefore, the first side of the fire tetrahedron (**FIGURE 3**) is an oxidizing agent that permits the fuel to burn.

The fuel is the material that oxidized. Since the fuel becomes chemically charged by the oxidizing process, it is a reducing agent. This makes the second side of the tetrahedron. Fuels can be anything from elements (carbon, hydrogen, magnesium) to compounds (cellulose, wood, paper, gasoline, petroleum compounds).

Some mixtures of reducing agent and oxidizing agent remain stable under certain conditions. However, when there is some activation energy, a chain reaction is started, which causes combustion. The factor that can trigger this chemical reaction can be as simple as exposing the combination to light. Once the chain reaction begins, extinguishments must take place by interrupting the chain reaction.

Scientists have known for many years that certain chemicals act as excellent extinguishing agents. However, they were at a loss to explain how these chemicals actually accomplished extinguishments, given the triangle of the fire model. With the development of the tetrahedron model and the inclusion of the uninhibited chain reaction, a scientifically sound theory could be postulated. With this as the basis, the extinguishing capabilities of the halons and certain dry chemicals were possible.

The final side of the tetrahedron is temperature. The fact that temperature is used instead of heat is deliberate. Temperature is the quantity of the disordered energy, which is what initiates combustion. It is possible to have a high heat as indicated by a large reading of Btu and still not have combustion. The temperature is therefore the key ingredient and the one that influences the action of the tetrahedron.

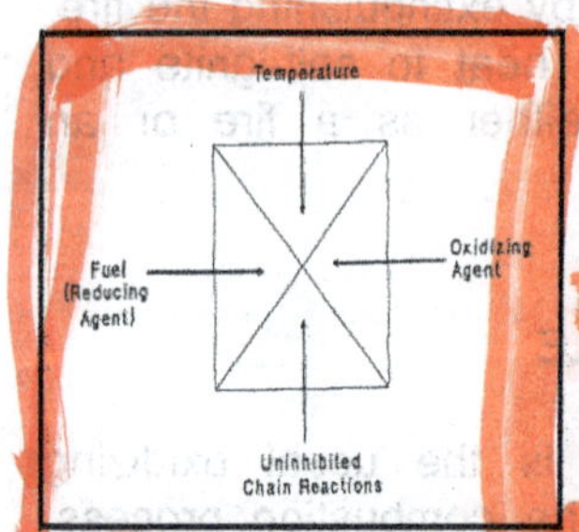

FIRE TETRAHEDRON

Flammability is the ability of a material of a material (liquid or gas) to generate enough concentration of combustible vapors under normal conditions to be ignited and produce a flame. It is necessary to have a proper fuel-to-air ratio (expressed as the percentage of fuel in air) to allow combustion. There is a range of fuel concentrations in air for each material that is optimal for the ignition and the sustenance of combustion. This is the Flammable Range. The lowest concentration of fuel in this range is the Lower Flammable Limit (LFL). Concentrations less than the LFL are not flammable because there is too little fuel – that is, the mixture is too "lean." The highest ratio that is flammable is the Upper Flammable Limit (UFL).

Concentrations greater than the UFL are not flammable because there is too much fuel displacing the oxygen (resulting in too little oxygen). This mixture is too "rich." Fuel concentrations between the LFL and the UFL are optimal for starting and sustaining fire. Example: the LFL for benzene is 1.3% (13,000 ppm), the UFL is 7.1% (71,000 ppm), and thus the flammable range is 1.3% to 7.1%.

A flammable material is considered highly combustible if it can burn at ambient temperatures. But a combustible material is not necessarily flammable, because it may not be easily ignited or the ignition maintained. For example, some pyrophoric materials will ignite at room temperature in the presence of a gas or vapor or when a slight friction or shock is applied.

It is important to note that the U.S. Department of Transportation (DOT), the Occupational Safety and Health Administration (OSHA), the National Institute for Occupational Safety and Health (NIOSH), and the National Fire Protection Association (NFPA) have established strict definitions for flammability based on the flash point of a material.

FLAMMABLE COMPOUNDS AND ELEMENTS	
Flammable Liquids	Flammable Solids
Aldehydes	Phosphorus
Ketones	Magnesium dust
Amines	Zirconium dust
Ethers	Titanium dust
Aliphatic hydrocarbons	Aluminum dust
Aromatic hydrocarbons	Zinc dust
Alcohols	
Nitroaliphatics	<u>Pyrophoric Liquids</u>
<u>Water-Reactive Flammable Solids</u>	Organometallic compounds
Potassium	Dimethyl zinc
Sodium	Tributyl aluminum
Lithium	

An **explosive** is a substance that undergoes a very rapid chemical transformation producing large amounts of gases and heat. The gases produced, for example, nitrogen, oxygen, carbon monoxide, carbon dioxide, and steam, due to the heat produced, rapidly expand at velocities exceeding the speed of sound. This creates both a shockwave (high pressure wave front) and noise.

Explosive gases/vapors exhibit an explosive range, which is the same as the flammable range. The upper explosive limit (UEL) and lower explosive limit (LEL) are the UFL and LFL but in confined areas. Most reference books list either explosive limits or flammable limits that are identical.

A **gas or vapor explosion** is a very rapid, violent release of energy. If combustion is extremely rapid large amounts of kinetic energy, heat, and gaseous products are released. The major factor contribution to the explosion is the confinement of a flammable material.

When vapors or gases cannot freely dissipate, they enter the combustion reaction more rapidly. Confinement also increases the energy associated with these molecules, which enhances the explosive process. Poorly ventilated buildings, sewers, drums, and bulk liquid containers are examples of places where potentially explosive atmospheres may exist.

There are several types of explosive hazards:

- **High or detonating**: chemical transformation occurs very rapidly with detonation rates as high as 4 miles per second. The rapidly expanding gas produces a shock wave which may be followed by combustion.

- **Primary high explosive**: detonating wave produced in an extremely short period of time. May be detonated by shock, heat, or friction. Examples are lead azide, mercury fulminate, and lead styphnate.

- **Secondary high explosive**: generally needs a booster to cause them to detonate. Relatively insensitive to shock, heat, or friction. Examples are tetryl, cyclonite, dynamite, and TNT.

- **Low or deflagrating**: Rate of deflagration up to 1000 feet per second. Generally combustion followed by a shock wave. Examples are smokeless powder, black power, and solid rocket fuel.

High or low does not indicate the explosion hazard (or power) but only the rate of chemical transformation. Explosions can occur as a result of reactions between many chemicals not ordinarily considered as explosives. Ammonium nitrate, a fertilizer, can explode under the right conditions. Alkali metals and water explode, as will water and peroxide salts. Picric acid and certain either compounds become highly explosive with age. Gases, vapors, and finely divided particulates, when confined, can also explode if an ignition source is present.

In summary, fires and explosions require fuel, air (oxygen), and an ignition source (heat). At a hazardous materials incident, the first two are not easily controlled. Consequently, while working on-site where a fire hazard may be present, the concentration of combustible gases in air must be monitored, and any potential source must be kept out of the area.

The most dangerous flammable substances:

- are easily ignited (e.g., pyrophorics).
- require little oxygen to support combustion.
- have low LFL/LEL and a wide Flammable/Explosive range.

Hazards related to fires and explosions cause:

- physical destruction due to shock waves, heat, and flying objects.
- initiation of secondary firs or creation of flammable conditions.
- release of toxic and corrosive compounds into the surrounding environment.

Corrosive Hazards

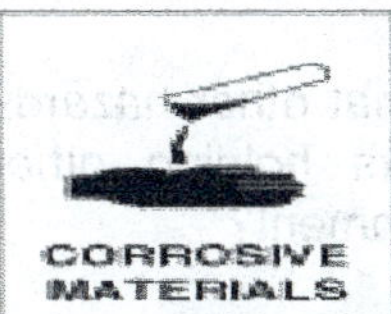

Corrosion is a process of material degradation. Upon contact, a corrosive material may destroy body tissues, metals, plastics, and other materials. Technically, corrosivity is the ability of material to increase the hydrogen ion or hydronium ion concentration of another material; it may have the potential to transfer electron pairs to or from itself or another substance. A corrosive agent is a reactive compound or element that produces a destructive chemical change in the material upon which it is acting. Common corrosives are the halogens, acids, and bases. Skin irritation and burns are typical results when the body contacts an acidic or basic material.

The corrosiveness of acids and bases can be compared on the basis of their ability to dissociate (form ions) in solution. Those that form the greatest number of hydrogen ions (H^+) are the strongest acids, while those that form the most hydroxide ions (OH^-) are the strongest bases. The H^+ ion concentration in solution is call pH. Strong acids have a low pH (many H^+ in solution) while strong bases have a high pH (few H^+ in solution; many OH^- in solution).

The pH scale ranges from 0 to 14 as follows:

< Increasing acidity   *Neutral*   *Increasing basicity>*

0   1   2   3   4   5   6   7   8   9   10   11   12   13   14

Measurements of pH are valuable because they can be quickly done on-site, providing immediate information on the corrosive hazard.

CORROSIVES

HALOGENS	ACIDS
Bromine	Acetic acid
Chlorine	Hydrochloric acid
Fluorine	Hydrofluoric acid
Iodine	Nitric acid
BASES (CAUSTICS)	Sulfuric acid
Potassium hydroxide	
Sodium hydroxide	

When dealing with corrosive materials in the field, it is imperative to determine:

- How toxic is the corrosive material? Is it an irritant or does it cause severe burns?
- What kind of structural damage does it do, and what other hazards occur? For example, will it destroy containers holding other hazardous materials, releasing them into the environment?

Chemical Reactivity

A **reactive material** is one that undergoes a chemical reaction under certain specified conditions. Generally, the term "reactive hazard" is used to refer to a substance that undergoes a violent or abnormal reaction in the presence of either water or normal ambient atmospheric conditions. Among this type of hazard are the pyrophoric liquids that will ignite in air at or below normal room temperature in the absence of added heat, shock, or friction, and the water-reactive flammable solids that will spontaneously combust upon contact with water.

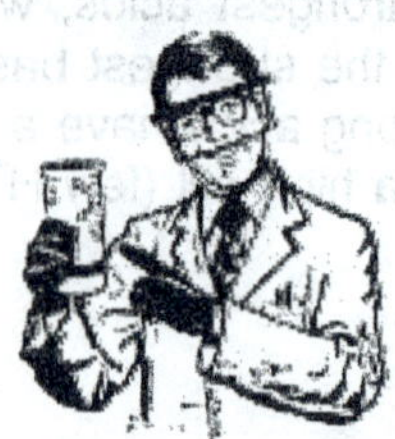

A **chemical reaction** is the interaction of two or more substances, resulting in chemical changes. Exothermic chemical reactions, which give off heat, can be the most dangerous. A separate source of heat is required to maintain endothermic chemical reactions. Removing the heat source stops the reaction.

Chemical reactions usually occur in one of the following ways:

- Combination   A + B   >   AB
- Decomposition   AB   >   A + B
- Single replacement   A + BC   >   B + AC
- Double replacement   AB + CD   >   AD + CB

The rate at which a chemical reaction occurs depends on the following factors:

- Surface area of reactants available at the reaction site – for example, a large chunk of coal is combustible, but coal dust is explosive.
- Physical state of reactant – solid, liquid, or gas
- Concentration of reactants
- Temperature
- Pressure
- Presence of a catalyst

If two or more hazardous materials remain in contact indefinitely without reaction, they are **compatible**. Incompatibility, however, does not necessarily indicate a hazard. For example, acids and bases (both corrosive) react to form salts and water, which may not be corrosive.

Many operations on waste or accident sites involve mixing or unavoidable contact between different hazardous materials. It is important to know ahead of time if such materials are compatible. If they are not, then any number of chemical reactions could occur. The results could range from the formation of an innocuous gas to a violent explosion.

The identity of unknown reactants must be determined by chemical analysis to establish compatibility. On the basis of their properties, a chemist then should be able to anticipate any chemical reactions resulting from mixing the reactants. Judging the compatibility of more than two reactants is very difficult; analysis should be performed on a one-to-one basis.

Response personnel who must determine compatibilities should refer to "A Method for Determining the Compatibility of Hazardous Wastes" (EPA

600/2-80-076), published by EPA's Office of Research and Development. Final decisions about compatibilities should only be made by an experienced chemist.

Sometimes the identity of a waste is impossible to ascertain due to money and time constraints. In this event, simple tests must be performed to determine the nature of the material or mixture. Tests such as pH, oxidation-reduction potential, and flashpoint are useful. In addition, very small amounts of the reactants may be carefully combined to determine compatibility.

If materials are compatible they may be stored together in bulk tanks or transferred to tank trucks for ultimate disposal. It is necessary, then, to establish the compatibility of the materials through analyses prior to bulking them. Compatibility information is also very important in evaluating an accident involving several different hazardous materials. The ultimate handling and treatment of the materials may be partially based on such information.

HAZARDS DUE TO CHEMICAL REACTIONS (INCOMPATIBILITIES)

Heat Generation	Acid and Water
Fire	Hydrogen Sulfide and Calcium Hypochlorite
Explosion	Picric Acid and Sodium Hydroxide
Toxic Gas or Vapor Production	Sulfuric Acid and Plastic
Flammable Gas or Vapor Production	Acid and Metal
Formation of a Substance with Greater Toxicity than the Reactants	Chlorine and Ammonia
Formation of Shock or Friction Sensitive Compounds	Peroxides and Organics OR Liquid Oxygen and Petroleum Products
Pressurization of Closed Vessels	Fire Extinguisher
Solubilization of Toxic Substances	Hydrochloric Acid and Chromium
Dispersal of Toxic Dusts and Mists	Sodium or Potassium Cyanide and Water or Acid Vapor
Violent Polymerization	Ammonia and Acrylonitrile

<u>Properties of Chemical Hazards</u>

Chemical compounds possess inherent properties that determine the type and degree of the hazard they represent. Evaluating risks of an incident depends on understanding these properties and their relationship to the environment.

The ability of a solid, liquid, gas, or vapor to dissolve in a solvent is **solubility**. An insoluble substance can be physically mixed or blended in a solvent for a short time but is unchanged with it finally separates. The solubility of a substance is independent of its density or specific gravity. The solubility of a material is important when determining its reactivity, dispersion, mitigation, and treatment. Solubility can be given in parts per million (ppm) or milligrams per liter (mg/L).

The **density** of a substance is its mass per unit volume, commonly expressed in grams per cubic centimeter (g/cc). The density of water is 1 g/cc since 1 cc has a mass of 1 g.

Specific gravity (SPG) is the ratio of the density of a substance (at a given temperature) to the density of water at the temperature of its maximum density (4°C). Numerically, SpG is equal to the density in g/cc, but is expressed as a pure number without units. If the SpG of a substance is greater than 1 (the SpG of water), it will sink in water. The substance will float on water if its SpG is less than 1. This is important when considering mitigation and treatment methods.

The **density of a gas or vapor** can be compared to the density of the ambient atmosphere. If the density of a vapor or gas is greater than that of the ambient air, then it will tend to settle to the lowest point. If vapor density is close to air density or lower, the vapor will tend to disperse in the atmosphere. Vapor density is given in relative terms similar to specific gravity. In settling, dense vapor creates two hazards. First, if the vapor displaces enough air to reduce the atmospheric concentration of oxygen below 16%, asphyxia may result. Second if the vapor is toxic, then inhalation problems predominate even if the atmosphere is not oxygen deficient. If a substance is explosive and very dense, the explosive hazard may be close to the ground rather than at the breathing zone (normal sampling heights).

The pressure exerted by a vapor against the sides of a closed container is called **vapor pressure**. It is temperature dependent. As temperature increases, so does the vapor pressure. Thus, more liquid evaporates or vaporizes. The lower the boiling point of the liquid, the greater the vapor pressure it will exert at a given temperature. Values for vapor pressure are most often given as millimeters of mercury (mm Hg) at a specific temperature.

The **boiling point** is the temperature at which a liquid changes to vapor – that is, it is the temperature where the pressure of the liquid equals atmospheric pressure. The opposite change in phases is the condensation point. Handbooks usually list temperatures as degrees Celsius (°C) or Fahrenheit (°F). A major consideration with toxic substances is how they enter the body. With high boiling-point liquids, the inhalation route is the most common and serious.

The temperature at which a solid changes phase to a liquid is the **melting point**. This temperature is also the freezing point, since a liquid can change phase to a solid. The proper terminology depends on the direction of the phase change. If a substance has been transported at a temperature that maintains a solid phase., then a change in temperature may cause the solid to melt. The particular substance may exhibit totally different properties depending on phase. One phase could be inert while the other highly reactive. Thus, it is imperative to recognize the possibility of a substance changing phase due to changes in the ambient temperature.

The minimum temperature at which a substance produces enough flammable vapors to ignite is its **flashpoint**. If the vapor does ignite, combustion can continue as long as the temperature remains at or above the flashpoint. The relative flammability of a substance is based on its flashpoint. An accepted relation between the two is:

Highly flammable:	Flashpoint less than 100°F
Moderately flammable:	Flashpoint greater than 100°F but less than 200°F
Relatively inflammable:	Flashpoint greater than 200°F

SAFETY HAZARDS

Safety is the condition of being secure from undergoing or causing hurt, injury, or loss. In this definition, safety requires a twofold posture – offensive and defensive. The offensive posture provides protection for actions one can control. The defensive posture is the awareness of factors or situations others may create. Care must be taken that actions to protect or reduce accident potentials for one person do not set up conditions ("booby traps") for subsequent accidents by other.

Kinetic/Mechanical

Generally referred to as "slip-trip-fall" type injuries, the kinetic/mechanical category includes "struck-by" injuries along with the "striking" injuries.

Workers must walk cautiously at the site to avoid tripping. Abandoned wastes usually are not kept neat and tidy. Train or other vehicle wrecks can produce debris that can increase the possibility of tripping. Problems at a hazardous waste site and an accident scene can be compounded by uneven terrain and mud, caused by rain or leaking chemicals.

Walking on drums is dangerous. Not only can they tip over, but they can be so corroded that they cannot support a person's weight. If it is necessary to walk over drums, place a piece of plywood over several drums and stand on this. This distributes the walker's weight over several drums. In some cases, a drum grappler can be used to move drums to a more accessible location.

Extra precautions must be taken if guardrails or railing are absent. The precautions generally include the use of a safety belt with a lifeline.

Electrical

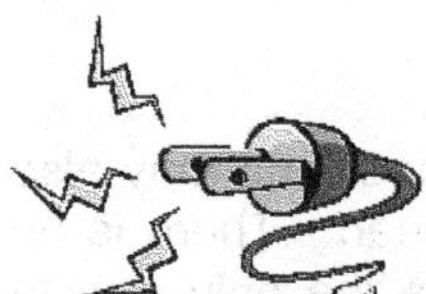

Electrical hazards can exist at accident sites because of downed power lines or improper use of electrical equipment. The presence of underground electric lines must be checked before any digging or excavating. When using cranes or material handlers, care must be taken that the machinery does not come in contact with any energized lines. There should be a 10-foot clearance between a crane and electric power lines unless the lines have been deenergized or an insulating barrier has been erected. Shock is the primary hazard from electrical tools. Although electrical shock may cause death, it can cause burns or falls that lead to injury.

Ways for protecting personnel from shock are:

- **Grounding equipment.** Grounding drains current, due to a short circuit, to earth. The ground wire is the third wire on three prong plugs. Equipment can also be grounded by a separate wire attached to the metal parts of equipment.

- **Using double-insulated tools**. These tools do not need to be grounded because they are: encased by a nonconductive material which is shatterproof, <u>or</u> have a layer of insulating material isolating the electrical components from a metal housing (used for more rugged design). This insulation is in addition to that found in regular tools. Double-insulated tools are identified by writing on the tool or by the symbol of a square with a square ([Y]).

- **Having overcurrent devices such as**: (1) fuses, which interrupt current by melting a fusible metal strip, or (2) circuit breakers, which operate by temperature change or magnetic difference.

  Overcurrent devices open the circuit automatically if the current is high from accidental ground, short circuit or overload. They should be selected based on type of equipment and capacity. A ground fault circuit interrupter (GFCI) device can be used to protect personnel and equipment. This device breaks a circuit when it detects low levels of current leaking to ground. It is fast-acting to keep the size of the current and its duration so low that it cannot produce serious injury. This device only operates on line-to-ground fault currents and not on line-to-line contact. It is commonly used on construction sites and in hospitals. Additionally, tools and flexible cords should be inspected for damage that could lead to shock. For more detailed information check the National Electrical Code (National Fire Protection Association Section 70).

Acoustic

Excessive acoustic energy can destroy the ability to hear and may also put stress on other parts of the body, including the heart. There is no cure for most effects of noise, therefore prevention is the only way to avoid health damage. The damage depends mainly on the intensity and length of exposure. The frequency or pitch can also have some effect, high-pitched sounds being more damaging than low-pitched ones.

Noise may tire out the inner ear, causing hearing loss. After a period of time off, hearing may be restored. Under some circumstances, the damage may become permanent because cells in the inner ear have been destroyed and can never be replaced or repaired. Permanent damage can be caused by long-term exposure to loud noise, or in some cases, by brief exposure to very loud noises (explosions, shock waves).

Although research on the effects of noise on other parts of the body is not complete, it appears that excessive noise can quicken the pulse rate, increase blood pressure, and narrow blood vessels. Over a long period of time, these may place an added burden on the heart.

Excessive noise may also put stress on other parts of the body by causing the abnormal secretion of hormones and tensing of muscles. Workers exposed to noise sometimes complain of nervousness, sleeplessness, and fatigue. Excessive noise exposure also can reduce job performance and may cause high rates of absenteeism.

OSHA regulation 29 CFR 1910.95 limits a worker's noise exposure to 90 decibels A weighted (dBA) for an 8-hour exposure. Time limits are shorter for higher noise levels. Decibel is the unit used in sound level measurements. Instruments generally are designed to use an A-weighted scale so that the instrument responds to the different sound frequencies in the same way as the human ear.

When daily noise exposure is composed of two or more periods of different noise levels, their combined effect should be considered, rather than the individual effect of each. If the sum – a time-weighted average (TWA) – of the following fractions $C_1/T1 + C_2/T_2 \ldots C_n/T_n$ exceeds 1, then the mixed exposure should be considered to exceed the limit value. C_n indicates the total time of exposure at a specific noise level, and T_n indicates the total time of exposure permitted at that level.

Recent rule making by OSHA requires a continued, effective hearing conservation program whenever worker noise exposures equal or exceed an 8-hour time-weighted average sound level (TWA) of 85 decibels measured on the A scale (dBA) or, equivalently, a dose of 50 percent.

The main elements of the hearing conservation program are:

- Monitoring of workers' exposures.

- An audiometric testing program for those exposed above an 85 dBA TWA. This requires a "baseline" audiogram for comparison and annual retesting to see if there is any hearing loss.

- Hearing protection <u>available</u> for those exposed to above 85 dBA TWA. If the TWA is above 90 dBA, or if it is above 85 dBA and the worker shows a permanent significant hearing loss, then hearing protection is <u>required</u> to be worn.

- Informing exposed workers about noise hazards (or effects) and the elements of a hearing conservation program.

The Environmental Protection Agency (EPA) recommends that, for an eight-hour work day, workers should not be exposed to noise levels above an 85 dBA TWA. EPA's goal is to reduce that level to 75 dBA. They also believe that individuals should not be exposed to a 70 dBA TWA for an entire 24-hour day.

<h2 align="center"><u>BIOLOGICAL HAZARDS</u></h2>

Animal bites/stings, contact with plants and microbes, and exposure to medical/infectious wastes are examples of biological hazards that response personnel may encounter.

Animal bites or stings are usually nuisances (localized swelling, itching, and minor pain) that can be handled by first aid treatments. The bites of certain snakes, lizards, spiders, and scorpions contain sufficient poison to warrant medical attention.

There are diseases that can be transmitted by animal bites. Examples are Rocky Mountain spotted fever (tick), rabies (mainly dogs, skunks, and foxes), malaria, and equine encephalitis (mosquito). The biggest hazard and most common cause of fatalities from animal bites – particularly bees, wasps, and spiders – is a sensitivity reaction. Anaphylactic shock due to stings can lead to severe reactions to the circulatory, respiratory, and central nervous system and it can also cause death.

Toxic effects from plants are generally due to ingestion of nuts, fruits, or leaves. Of more concern to response personnel are certain plants, including poison ivy, poison oak, and poison sumac, which produce adverse effects from direct contact.

The usual effect is dermatitis – inflammation of the skin. The protective clothing and decontamination procedures used for chemicals also reduce the exposure risk from the plant toxins. Cleaning the skin thoroughly with soap and water after contact will reduce the risk.

Another source of infection for response workers is poor sanitation. Waterborne and foodborne diseases can be a problem if adequate precautions are not taken. Examples of waterborne diseases are cholera, typhoid fever, viral hepatitis, salmonellosis, bacillary dysentery, and amebic dysentery. In an emergency response related to a disaster, water supplies may be affected. The source of water for a long-term remedial action is also important. In some locations, it may be necessary to transport water and food to the site. They must be handled properly and come from an uncontaminated source.

The response team must also avoid creating any sanitation problems by making sure that properly designed lavatory facilities are available at the worksite.

Microbial hazards can occur when the materials the workers are handling have biological as well as chemical contamination. This can be a problem is a chemical spill is into or mixed with sewage. Most bacteria that affect humans prefer a neutral environment (pH 7). Thus an extremely acid or alkaline environment would destroy or inhibit bacterial growth. However, during neutralization, the environment could become more conducive to bacteria growth. In these situations, the normal decontamination procedures will usually alleviate the problem.

Medical/infectious wastes include **bloodborne pathogens**, which are regulated by OSHA 29 CFR 1910.1030. This standard specifically addresses proper engineering controls, work practices, and personal protective equipment to reduce the risk of contact with bloodborne pathogens.

<u>**RADIATION HAZARDS**</u>

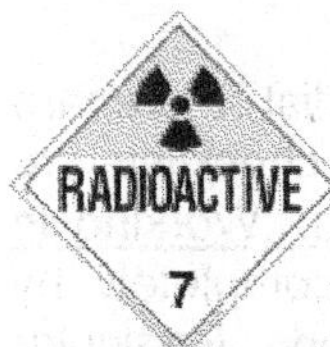

Radioactive materials that may be encountered at a site can emit three types of harmful radiation: alpha particles, beta particles, and gamma waves. All three forms harm living organisms by imparting energy which ionizes molecules in the cells. Therefore, the three are referred to as ionizing radiation. Ionization may upset the normal cellular function causing cell dysfunction or death.

An alpha particle is positively charged. The beta is an electron possessing a negative charge. Both particles have mass and energy. Both are emitted from the nucleus. They travel short distances in material before interactions with the material causes them to lose their energy. The outer layers of the skin and clothing generally protect against these particles. Therefore, they are considered hazardous primarily when they enter the body through inhalation or ingestion.

Gamma radiation is pure electromagnetic energy and is wave-like rather than particulate. Gamma waves pass through all materials to some degree. Clothing, including protective gear, will not prevent gamma radiation from interacting with body tissue.

Unlike many hazardous substances that possess certain properties which can alert response personnel to over-exposures (odor, irritation, or taste), radiation has no such warning properties. Therefore, preventing radiation material from entering the body or protecting against external radiation is the best protection. As with biological and chemical hazards, the use of respiratory and personnel protective equipment, coupled with scrupulous personal hygiene, will afford good protection against radioactive particulates.

CONFINED SPACE HAZARDS

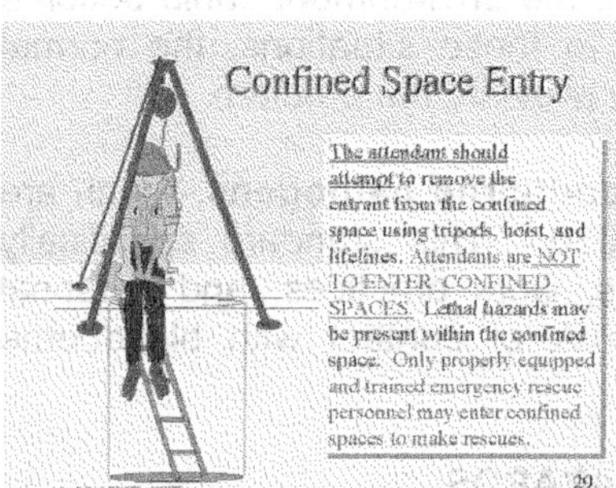

NIOSH defines a **confined space** as any space which by design has limited openings for entry and exit; unfavorable natural ventilation which could contain or produce dangerous air contaminants, and which is not intended for continuous worker occupancy. Examples of confined spaces would include storage tanks, holds of ships, process vessels, pits, silos, boilers, ventilation and exhaust ducts, sewers, tunnels, underground utility vaults, and pipelines.

The NIOSH classifications of confined spaces use a checklist to prepare for and carry out confined space operations safely. These checklists are found in NIOSH's "Criteria for a Recommended Standard…Working in Confined Spaces." This document should be studied completely by anyone responsible for the oversight of confined space work. Particular professional judgement, skill, and experience is required to conduct confined space operations safely. All items listed on the checklist must be in place and utilized in order to assure worker health and safety during the most dangerous hazardous materials work activity that of confined space work.

While complete data is not available, working in confined spaces is recognized as the most dangerous type of work involving hazardous materials. The very nature of a confined space increases the likelihood of encountering a toxic atmosphere because the confined space encourages the accumulation of gases and vapor. A very high rate of accidents involving worker fatalities is associated with confined spaces. Again, while complete data is impossible to obtain, studies have suggested that as many as two-thirds of all confined space fatalities are would-be rescuers. For every worker who initially is overcome and eventually dies as a result of confined space exposure, perhaps two would-be rescuers are succumbing also. The main reason that this occurs is that workers do not recognize the hazard presented by the confined space.

A closed building, or room, are examples of confined spaces that response personnel may encounter. Procedures for entry into a confined space are very similar to entry into a site. Because of poor ventilation, high concentrations of gases or vapors are more likely to exist in a confined space than at an open site. Also, certain confined spaces may contain hazardous materials. For example, hydrogen sulfide and methane are often in sewers. Also a large amount of organic material in an enclosed space can combine with oxygen in the surrounding air to produce an oxygen deficient atmosphere.

Besides the problem with possible high concentration of gases or vapors, confined spaces also present an entrance and exit problem. Most of the spaces mentioned earlier have only small openings for entry and exit. This can interfere with use of equipment like self-contained breathing apparatus (SCBA). In some cases an airline respirator may have to be used in place of an SCBA. Because of this problem, and in case a worker is injured, a lifeline is often attached to the worker to aid in pulling him out. That way rescuers would not have to enter the space. A lifeline is especially important in spaces where access is through an opening in the top of the space.

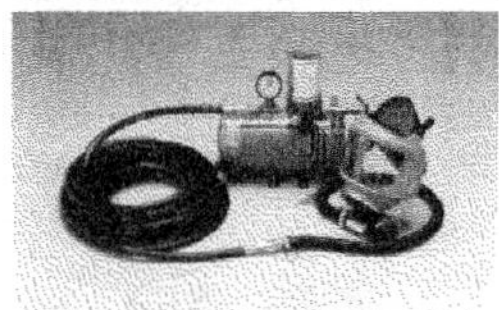

Lockout, blocking, or equivalent measures may be needed to ensure that deactivated systems are not reactivated at inopportune times (**FIGURE 4**). These procedures are usually used when someone is working on or around equipment that could cause injury if it is accidentally turned on.

The general procedure is to turn off the equipment at a point where it can be locked so that the equipment cannot be turned on. An example is the main power disconnect on a fuse box. Most boxes have a tab and hole where a lock can be placed so the switch cannot be turned back on. For piping systems, not only can the valve be turned off, but the pipes can be disconnected or a blank – a flat plate inserted in the pipeline. These two methods may be used in lieu of actually locking a valve. The advantage of using an actual lock is that only one person has a key; therefore, only he can reactive the equipment after he is done with repair work. In some cases, there may be several workers,, each using a different lock on a switch so that all locks have to be removed before equipment can be used.

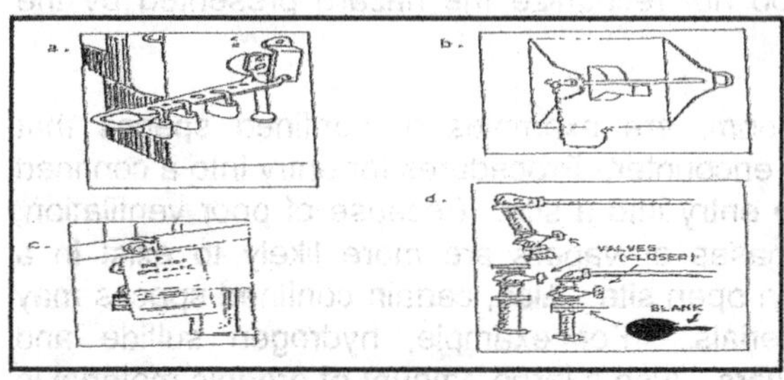

LOCKOUT, BLOCKING, AND TAGGING (a) MULTIPLE LOCKS; (b) BLOCK ON SWITCH; (c) TAG; (d) DISCONNECTING AND "BLANKING" PIPELINE

MEDICAL EMERGENCIES

Hazardous material environments pose unique health hazards for personnel. A medical program is necessary to assess and monitor the workers' health and fitness both prior to work and during the course of work activities. It is important for personnel to recognize medical emergencies and to be trained on emergency procedures and treatment.

Heat Stress

The human body is designed to function at a certain internal temperature. When metabolism or external sources (fire, hot summer day) cause the body temperature to rise, the body seeks to protect itself by triggering cooling mechanisms. Excess heat is dissipated by two means:

- Changes in blood flow to dissipate heat by convection, which can be seen as "flushing" or reddening of the skin in extreme cases.

- Perspiration, the release of water through skin and sweat glands. While working in hot environments, evaporation of perspiration is the primary cooling mechanism.

Protective clothing worn to guard against chemical contact effectively stops the evaporation of perspiration. Thus the use of protective clothing increases heat stress problems.

The major disorders due to heat stress are heat cramps, heat exhaustion, and heat stroke. **Heat cramps** are painful spasms which occur in the skeletal muscles of workers who sweat profusely in the heat and drink large quantities of water, but fail to replace the body's lost salts or electrolytes. Drinking water while continuing to lose salt tends to dilute the body's extracellular fluids. Soon water seeps by osmosis into active muscles and causes pain. Muscles fatigued from work are usually most susceptible to cramps.

Heat exhaustion is characterized by extreme weakness or fatigue, dizziness, nausea, and headache. In serious cases, a person may vomit or lose consciousness. The skin is clammy and moist, complexion pale or flushed, and body temperature normal or slightly higher than normal. Treatment is rest in a cool place and replacement of body water lost by perspiration. Mild cases may recover spontaneously with this treatment; severe cases may require care for several days. There are no permanent effects.

Heat stroke is a very serious condition caused by the breakdown of the body's heat regulating mechanism. The skin is very dry and got with a red, mottled or bluish appearance. Unconsciousness, mental confusion, or convulsions may occur. Without quick and adequate treatment, the result can be death or permanent brain damage. Get medical assistance quickly! As first aid treatment, the person should be moved to a cool place. Body heat should be reduced artificially, but not too rapidly, by soaking the person's clothes with water and fanning them.

Steps that can be taken to reduce heat stress are:

- Acclimatize the body. Allow a period of adjustment to make further heat exposure endurable. It is recommended that a new worker start at 50% of the anticipated total work load for the first day and increase the work load gradually each succeeding day for about a week. Acclimatization can be "lost" if a worker is away from the heat for two weeks.

- Drink more liquids to replace body water lost during sweating.

- Rest frequently.

- Increase salt consumption. Sweat is mostly water with smaller amounts of sodium and potassium salts. Replacement fluids should be similar in composition. Thus, salt tablets usually are not necessary and can be harmful. It is better to increase salt on food or drink commercially available preparations that provide the proper balance of water and salts.

- Wear personal cooling devices. There are two basic designs; units with pockets for holding frozen packets and units that circulate a cooling fluid from a reservoir through tubes to different parts of the body. Both designs can be in the form of a vest, jacket, or coverall. Some circulating units also have a cap for cooling the head.

- Wear supplied air suits or respirators that are equipped with a vortex tube that either cools or warms the air being supplied. The vortex tube is not used with self-contained breathing apparatus because it uses large amounts of compressed air during operation.

- Wear cotton long underwear under chemical protective clothing. The cotton will absorb perspiration and will hold it close to the skin. This will provide the body with the maximum cooling available from the limited evaporation that takes place beneath chemical resistant clothing. It also allows for rapid cooling of the body when the protective clothing is removed.

There are instruments that measure air temperature, radiant heat, and humidity to give a heat index. The National Institute for Occupational Safety and Health (NIOSH), American Conference of Governmental Industrial Hygienists (ACGIH), and other groups use this index in their guidelines on heat stress. However, these guidelines are usually valid only for acclimatized personnel wearing light summer clothing and not chemical resistant or insulating protective gear.

Cold Exposure

Cold temperatures can also cause medical problems. The severe effects are frostbite and hypothermia.

Frostbite is the most common injury resulting from exposure to cold. The extremities of the body are most often affected. The signs of frostbite are: the skin turns white or grayish-yellow, pain is sometimes felt early but subsides later (often there is no pain), and the affected part feels intensely cold and numb.

Standard first aid for frostbite includes getting the victim to a warm shelter. Put frozen parts in warm water (100-105°F) but not hot water. Handle parts gently and do not rub or massage them. If toes and fingers are affected, put dry, sterile gauze between them after warming them. Loosely bandage the injured parts. If the part has been thawed and refrozen rewarm it at room temperature.

Hypothermia is characterized by shivering, numbness, drowsiness, muscular weakness and a low internal body temperature when the body feels warm externally. This can lead to unconsciousness and death. In the case of hypothermia, professional medical care should be sought immediately. A victim should be taken out of the cold and into dry clothing. The body should be warmed slowly.

Medical Surveillance

Medical surveillance is important in two ways. First, since response workers are handling 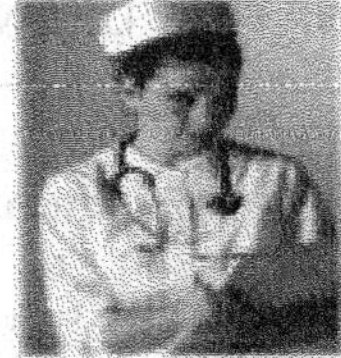 materials that can damage their bodies, they must be checked to determine if any damage is occurring. There are medical tests for determining if a worker has too much of a chemical in their system. For example, blood tests can detect lead and carbon monoxide, urine tests can detect arsenic, and there are tests to determine if the liver is functioning properly. Exhaled air and hair and nail clippings can also be analyzed for the presence of chemicals. Workers showing an abnormal amount of chemical in their systems should be removed from their assignments or have their operating procedures reevaluated.

The second reason for medical surveillance is to ensure that the worker is capable of doing the job. Using respiratory protection attains the pulmonary system. OSHA General Industry Standard 29 CFR 1910.134(b)(10) states that "Persons should not be assigned to tasks requiring use of respirators unless it has been determined that they are physically able to perform the work and use the equipment." Heat stress can be a problem for workers wearing protective clothing. Thus, in some situations, it would be advisable to check workers for symptoms of heat stress.

Medical Emergencies and First Aid

OSHA Construction Industry Standard 29 CFR 1926.50 – Medical Services and First Aid requires that:

- Medical personnel be available for advice and consultation on matters of occupational health.

- Prior to start of the project, provisions be made for prompt medical attention in case of serious injury.

- At least one and preferably more persons at the worksite be trained in first aid. The American Red Cross, some insurance carriers, local safety councils, and other organizations provide acceptable training.

- First aid supplies approved by a consulting physician be readily available. The supplies should be in sanitary and weatherproof containers with individually sealed packages for material such as

- gauze, bandages, and dressings that must be sterile.

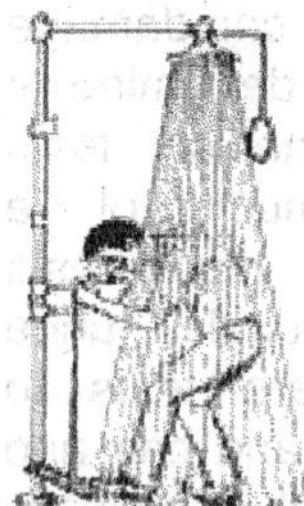

COMBINATION DRENCH SHOWER AND EYEWASH

- Proper equipment be provided for prompt transportation of an injured person to a physician or hospital, or a communication system for contacting necessary ambulance service.

- The telephone numbers of the physicians, hospitals, or ambulances be conspicuously posted.

Medical assistance will probably be available at an emergency response such as a truck or train wreck. It is important to remember that first aid is immediate temporary treatment given in the event of accident or illness before the doctor arrives. Some states have laws establishing limits on first aid given by the lay person. Trained employees should understand where first aid ends and professional medical treatment begins.

Additionally, OSHA's Medical Services and First Aid Standard (29 CFR 1910.151) for general industry require that the areas where workers may be exposed to splashes of corrosive materials should have facilities for flushing the chemicals out of eyes and from the body. If a decontamination line has been set up, it may provide the protection needed. Otherwise, additional facilities will be needed. For example, eyewashes and drench showers may be necessary in such areas as laboratories, solvent-dispensing areas, and battery recharging stations where harmful material may be splashed in the eyes or on the skin. Such units can be hooked to a water line or may be portable with a self-contained water supply. It is important to remove chemicals from the body immediately even if protective clothing is worn because the clothing does not stop penetration or permeation of all chemicals.

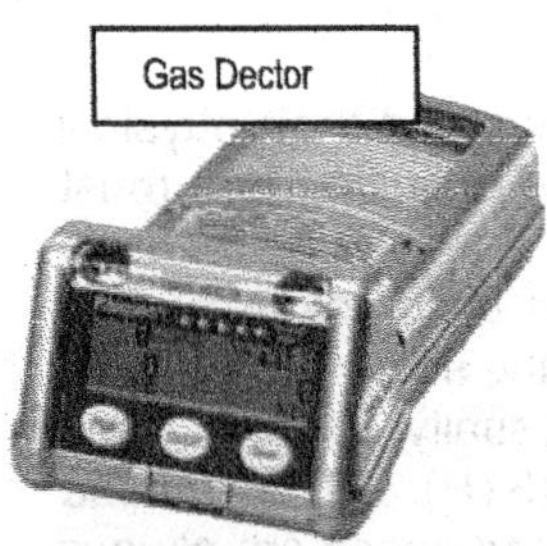

Gases, by the definition of the word itself, denote chaos. Whether by looking at the way they can move or how they physically react, gases represent a physical state of hazardous materials that requires specific attention. For centuries, early researchers understood the basic physical properties of liquids or solids, but vapors or "airs" remained misunderstood or generally unknown. Scientists realized that the air around them did have specific properties, but since most gases are invisible, little study was made. Until the eighteenth century, bad air, such as from swamps (methane, then known as marsh gas), was tested as a health hazard. Today, we still use the term malaria to denote a medical condition although the word was derived from the Italian language and literally means "bad air". Not until the experiments of Allesandro Volta (the creator of the first true battery), was marsh gas treated with scientific respect.

Further experimentation was done isolating specific gases in the atmosphere. With the successes of Priestly (oxygen, 1771) and Cavendish (hydrogen, 1766), science began to understand that not only was ambient air comprised of more than one gas, but also gases came from other sources and represented specific hazards. Priestly for example, suspended objects in the "fixed air" (carbon dioxide) above beer vats. His subjects included mice, which died, and candles, which went out, thus giving the first evidence of one of the prime hazards of gases—asphyxiation. One workplace that has characteristically represented a hazardous atmosphere and indeed still does is mines, especially coal mines. Here the inherent dangers of firedamp and afterdamp are still prevalent today.

It is critical for the complete study of hazardous materials to include a chapter on gases and vapors and how to detect their presence through air monitoring. The use and production of gases in the post-Industrial Revolution society is manifold. Not only mines, but also almost all major industrial processes such petrol-chemicals and computer manufacturers rely upon gases for production. Naturally produced gases such as methane and hydrogen sulfide also pose a problem as well as gases found in waste sites, drums, confined spaces, sewage treatment, chemical manufacturing, and agriculture. Gases and vapors, both man-made and natural represent a health hazard and require air monitoring. Due to the large variety of gases present in our society, it is beyond the scope of this chapter to explain how all may react. We will, however, understand how gases "work" where they may accumulate, and how their presence is determined in order to make the workplace safer and to protect human life.

In order to work with gases, it is important to understand their physical state and nature of movement. To understand the definition one must also recognize the three hazards that gases pose. First, a gas tends to occupy the space of its container. Thus, if the gas becomes free of its container, it will continue to expand until it reaches the same pressure as the ambient atmosphere. This is why gases usually expand upon release at standard temperature and pressure (STP). The second hazard described in this definition is that manufactured gases are always in some sort of container, such as a cylinder. With a change in the physical characteristics of the gas, the cylinder can rupture or explode, becoming a missile hazard. Finally, each gas has a vapor density in relation to the normal atmosphere. Many gases such as hydrogen, methane, neon, and other gases will rise into the atmosphere and disperse. Other gases are heavier than air and will sink and collect in low spots, often taking time to disperse. An example of this is chlorine. It is a heavy, dense gas that dissipates slowly under normal conditions. For this reason it was used as the first major poison gas in April of 1915 in World War I. Soldiers exposed to the gas sought refuge out of the trenches while their colleagues choked to death a few feet below them in the bottom of shell holes and trenches.

GAS LAWS

Although gases were discussed previously, it is important to emphasize the specific physical characteristics of gases as they relate to hazardous materials response. In most cases, gases are stored and transported under pressure in containers. By altering the physical factors that act upon gases, such as excessive pressure or heat, they can become unstable. Since these conditions may arise even under normal atmospheric conditions, gases must be treated with a high level of respect. There is a reason why in transportation gases (DOT class 2) are considered the second highest hazard after explosives (DOT class 1). They can rise, sink, flow, burn, explode, asphyxiate, poison, and corrode people and equipment.

Before going further into the physical hazards of a gas, it is important to understand the basic properties of gases. Understanding gases is dependent upon the relationship between the volume of a gas, its temperature and pressure. These principles are validated through the following mathematical equations. Other factors are used to determine mass and volume of gasses, but the scope of this section is to give the reader the understanding that gases are primarily affected by changes in temperature, pressure, and/or volume. The result of any significant change in these conditions may lead to container failure, one of the driving themes of this chapter.

The first of the gas laws to be demonstrated is Boyle's law, named after its creator, Robert Boyle. This law states that the volume of a gas varies inversely with pressure when temperature is a constant. Thus:

$$P \times V = constant$$
$$P_1 \times V_1 = P_2 \times V_2$$

In this formula, P and V denote pressure and volume. P_1 and V_1 are the initial pressure and volume and P_2 and V_2 are the final values for pressure and volume. For example, if you want to know what volume 100 cubic feet (100 ft^3) of a random gas occupies if its pressure is changed from 15 to 250 psia with temperature remaining fixed, Boyle's law can thus read:

$$V_2 = 100 \text{ ft}^3 \times \frac{15 \text{ psia}}{250 \text{ psia}} = 6 \text{ ft}^3$$

The second gas law to be determined was by the French scientist Jacques Charles. Charles's law demonstrates that if pressure is a constant, then volume increases with an increase in temperature. A simple example is the energy force behind a hot air balloon. Thus, if a gas sample is compared at a constant pressure but different temperatures and volumes. Charles's law can be demonstrated as follows:

$$V_1 = V_2 \text{ or } V_1 = T_1$$
$$T_1 = T_2 \qquad V_2\ T_2$$

In these formulas, V and T denote volume and temperature (absolute). V_1 and T_1 denote initial volume and temperature, and V_2 and T_2 denote final volume and temperature. Absolute temperature, or Kelvin (K) must be used to factor the temperature. [0 K = -273.15°C and 0°C= 273.15K]. 273.15 K]. Thus, if a 250 cubic millimeter plastic bag of a random gas is heated from 25°C to 40°C, the final volume after warming can be determined as follows:

$$V_1 = 250 \text{ cm}^3$$
$$T_1 = 25°C \text{ or } 298.15K$$
$$T_2 = 40°C \text{ or } 313.15K$$

Substituting the above values for V_2, the following applies:

$$250 \text{ cm}^3 = V_2$$
$$298.15 \qquad 313.15$$

or,

$$V_2 = \frac{313.15}{298.15} \times 250 \text{ cm}^3 = 262 \text{ cm}^3$$

When neither temperature of pressure is constant both Boyle's law and Charles's law can be combined into the following formula known as the Combined Gas law:

$$V_1 = T_1 \times P_2$$
$$V_2 \quad T_2 P_1$$

The final consideration of these laws is that the volume of a gas may be forced to remain constant while the other factors that drive Boyle's law and Charles's law change. In other words, the gas is in a container such as a metal cylinder. In this case the values of V_1 and V_2 remain the same. As the gas is heated, the pressure increases. This is referred to as Amonton's law

$$P_1 = P_2$$
$$T_1 \quad T_2$$

When the temperature of a cylinder is increased significantly (such as in a fire), the cylinder may rupture or explode.

DETECTION OF GASES

The amount of a gas that may adversely affect us may be extremely small. Arsine gas, for example, has an immediately dangerous to life and health (IDLH) of approximately 3 ppm. Gases may be invisible, colorless, or odorless. Never should your sense of smell be used to find a gas. Never should an environment be judged "clean" because it looks clean. The detection of gases present in an environment shall always be done with correctly calibrated instruments. Gases can pose a significant hazard to your health in various manners. Thus, the monitoring of an atmosphere can reduce your risk of exposure to a gas. To perform this function, a series of different monitors are used. Keep in mind there is no such thing as a universal gas monitor that performs all functions required to completely analyze a test atmosphere. This chapter describes each monitor and it purpose.

There are various manufacturers and models of air monitoring equipment on the market. Some models may perform more than one function, test for different levels, or test for a variety of gases, but all work in the same manner to identify contaminants in the atmosphere.

When detecting gases, some groups such as public agencies may have to take steps to identify a completely unknown atmosphere because the source could be almost anything. In other situations, such as in a factory, a hazardous materials response team may know exactly what has been released or at least be able to narrow down the potential release due to knowing what is present at their facility and where it is. In other words, if you know what is present because it is the only possible chemical present, then air monitoring may be done only to confirm the presence of that material. Do not waste time in running tests for unknown gases. Before or even during air monitoring procedures, responders can be on the lookout for other methods of identification such as labeling and placarding.

The use of monitoring equipment not only protects the health and safety of the individual but allows waste workers and responders in the hazardous materials field to establish other factors such as selecting the proper level of personal protection equipment, establishing control zones and evacuation areas, defining a decontamination corridor, assessing the potential health effects of exposure, and determining the need for specific medical monitoring. Air monitoring is a continuous, ongoing process. Air monitoring shall be done not only upon first entry or investigation of an environment, but on a regular basis throughout any operation. Ongoing air monitoring allows for changes in the atmosphere due to heating or cooling during the day, movement due to natural or forced ventilation, the movement of toxic materials themselves, and any other situation that may alter atmospheric conditions.

In most cases, detection is made using hand-held, direct-reading instruments. The choice of a specific model is up to the individual, but any instrument used should be portable and rugged, easy to operate under field conditions, intrinsically safe (not a spark hazard), and produce reliable and useful results. Waste workers and responders using air-monitoring equipment shall be trained on how to use them properly and correctly analyze their results. Never should an individual be expected to learn an instrument by using it as he or she "goes along." Everybody should have a strong level of confidence not only in the accuracy of their equipment, but also in their ability to correctly use it and analyze data.

This chapter describes the sequence to be used by members of a properly trained cleanup or response team who determine atmospheric hazards. In other words, use a step-by-step process to confirm the presence of a hazardous situation involving oxygen levels and/or the presence of gas hazards. Remember, you are there to rapidly determine the presence or absence of atmospheric hazards and to contain and control the release. Further testing may require the specialties of an industrial hygienist.

An industrial hygienist uses the same or similar tools described in this chapter, but does so in a more precise manner. This does not mean that results in the field are faulty. Those quickly obtained results tell whether a chemical is present and to what extent atmospheric contamination can be expected. For example, a properly trained waste worker or responder may test a storage tank for oxygen deficiency or the presence of a combustible gas. An example of the work of industrial hygienists is working with "sick buildings" or "sick rooms." In this situation, precise readings and levels must be determined to find out exactly what is present and exactly where the source is. In sick rooms or buildings it is not a spill or release of a chemical as is common with hazardous materials incidents, but dealing with offgassing from consumer articles such as carpet, chairs, and plastics. An industrial hygienist may also have to research the previous use of the land and work/life habits of involved personnel to further determine what my be causing the complaint.

THE SEQUENCE OF AIR MONITORING

As mentioned, there is no such thing as a universal gas detector. To properly determine the atmospheric conditions of a space, tank, cylinder, or area, various types of monitors are required. The following is the suggested thought process to be followed in testing an atmosphere:

- First, if radioactive materials are known or suspected in the test atmosphere, the use of radiation monitors is required. This action is more the exception than the rule due to the relative rarity of incidents involving radioactive materials.

- Thus, an oxygen indicator is generally used first, primarily in areas that may be oxygen deficient, such as a confined space.

- Next, a combustible gas indicator (CGI) is used to detect the presence of combustible gases or vapors.

- A flame ionization detector (FID) is used to detect organic gases and vapors. This device may include a gas chromatograph. In many situations, the use of this device is optional.

- An ultraviolet photoionizaton detector (PID) is used to detect organic and some inorganic gases and vapors. Like an FID, the use of this device may be considered optional.

- Finally, a system of colorimetric indicator tubes is used to identify specific gases.

THE USE OF AIR MONITORING EQUIPMENT

Oxygen Meters

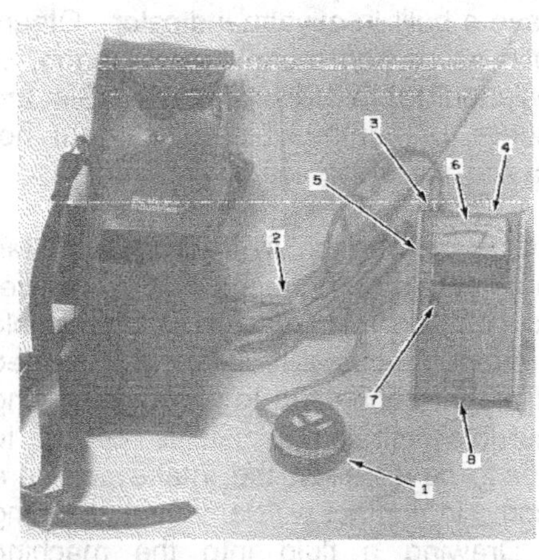

The first monitor that should be used is the oxygen meter unless the presence of radioactive material is known or suspected, especially in a situation where there is the possibility of oxygen deficiency or oxygen enrichment such as a confined space. Oxygen meters work on the principle of allowing oxygen to diffuse into a detector cell and measuring a chemical reaction establishing a current between two electrolyte cells. The normal percentage of oxygen in the atmosphere is approximately 21% at sea level. According to the Occupational Safety and Health Administration (OSHA), any atmosphere less than 19.5% oxygen is considered oxygen deficient and any atmosphere more than 23.5% oxygen is considered oxygen enriched and thus an increased fire hazard. Oxygen meters may be used to determine the type of respiratory protection required, the risk of combustion, and if there may be variation on other instruments used such as a combustible gas indicator. Many models do not work accurately in less than 16% oxygen. Oxygen meters are straightforward instruments that have a visual readout and an audible warning that alarms when the oxygen levels drops below 19.5% or rises above

23.5%. Like all instruments they require calibration and zeroing before use. This setting should be done in a normal oxygen level atmosphere before the instrument is exposed to the test atmosphere. The accuracy of an oxygen indicator may be affected by changes in altitude or barometric pressure or the presence of certain gases such as ozone or carbon dioxide, which can damage the detector cell.

COMBUSTIBLE GAS INDICATORS

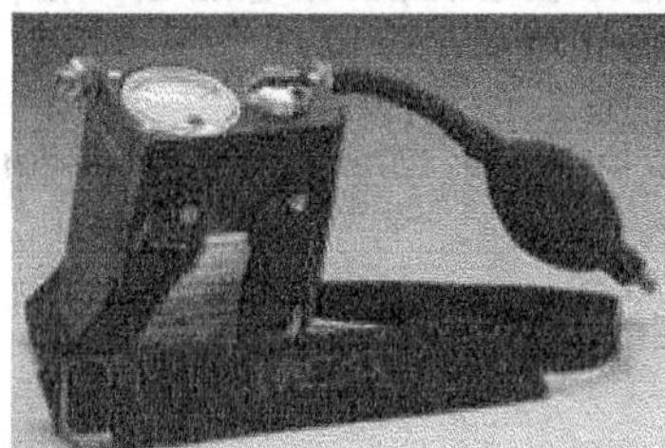

The second instrument to be used is a combustible gas indicator (CGI). The market for these instruments is large and so too is the variety. Keep in mind that considerations discussed in choosing which instrument is right for the task in mind. If the device is complicated, many people simply won't use it. Many CGIs are considered multigas detectors and may have a built-in oxygen indicator. Others may detect specific gases such as carbon monoxide, methane, or hydrogen sulfide. If not designed for a specific gas, CGIs are designed to detect the presence of combustible gases, but not determine what combustible gas or gases are actually present.

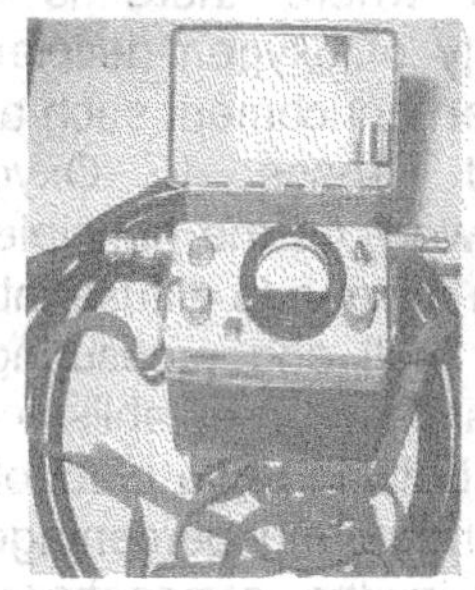

Many CGI'S operate on this principle: A fan draws in a sample of the test atmosphere over a heated catalytic filament. If a combustible gas is present, electrical resistance is created on one filament connected to a circuit causing a measurable imbalance. It is critical to remember to never allow the intake port of a CGI to come in contact with any fluid including water. Drawing a fluid into the machine compromises the device and requires extensive (and expensive) repairs. A combusition indicatior is designed to give a visual and audible alarm usually at 10% of the lower explosive limit (LEL). This allows for a large safety factor due to variables in detecting the combustible gas. These variables include an oxygen-deficient atmosphere; the type of calibration gas (such as hexane or methane) used in the CGI itself, variation in temperature, and the presence of interfering materials such as lead, sulfur, silicones, hydrogen chloride, and hydrogen fluoride. When a CGI alarms, the machine is telling you of an oxygen-deficient atmosphere or that a combustible gas is present. The CGI does not determine what the combustible gas is unless the machine is a multigas detector calibrated for specific gases. In this situation the device can warn of the presence of gases such as carbon monoxide or hydrogen sulfide if it is designed to do so. As with all monitors, a CGI requires proper calibration and zeroing before each use and recalibration with the test gas in a periodic manner.

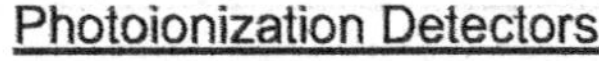

Photoionization Detectors

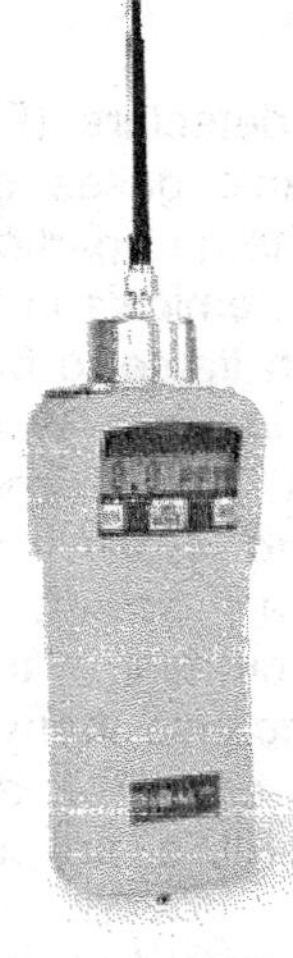

Photoionization detectors (PIDs) are designed to detect relatively low concentrations of contaminants usually in the range of 0.1 to 2000 ppm. They are efficient in detecting aromatic hydrocarbons such as benzene, toluene, xylene, and vinyl chloride. They work by drawing a sample of the test atmosphere into a chamber with an ultraviolet (UV) lamp. The UV light breaks down the sample by displacing electrons and measures the energy required to do so. This process is called the *ionization potential* (IP) and each chemical compound has a unique IP. Thus, it is possible to determine an actual gas by reading the IP off the PID and comparing it to known levels of gases. One reference source is the NIOSH *Pocket Guide to Hazardous Materials,* which lists the IP for each compound. Another factor with the PID is that there is a variety of UV lamps with different electron volts (eV) capabilities. Ionization potential is measured in electron volts, so the correct lamp must be used to determine the gas. The contaminant gas must have an IP less than the eV capacity of the UV lamp. One of the key considerations for this device is that it must be properly calibrated and accurately spanned before use to ensure the proper IP is determined, which is best determined by consulting the manufacturer's date tables.

The PID strap allows the body of the machine to be hung off the shoulder while the wand is used to collect the sample. PID's work well with small concentrations, but high concentrations may cause false low readings. Other variable factors include water vapor (humidity), nonionizing gases, diesel exhaust, smoke, soil, and a dirty UV lamp. Although a PID can detect many ionizing materials at low levels, they do not detect everything. For example, they cannot detect methane; therefore they are used in conjunction with the other instruments.

Example ionization potentials

Chemical	IP (eV)	Chemical	IP (eV)
Acetone	9.69	Ethylene oxide	10.56
Ammonia	10.18	Hydrogen peroxide	10.54
Carbon dioxide	13.77	Toluene	8.82
Chlorine	11.48	Vinyl chloride	9.99

Flame Ionization Detectors

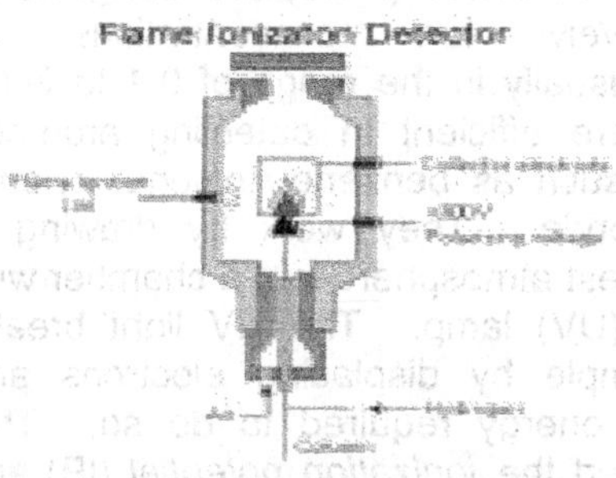

Flame ionization detectors (FID) detect many organic gases and vapors by using charged particles or ions to detect chemicals in the air and a hydrogen flame to burn organic materials in air. As the test contaminant is burned, positively charged ions are produced and a current is generated. This current is then measured on a scale relative to a calibrant gas. Because many of the capabilities of an FID are overlapped by those of a PID, and because of their high cost and maintenance, FID's are not commonly used except by specialized hazardous materials teams. If they are used however, they do have an advantage over PIDs in that in the survey mode, they can read 0 to 1,000 ppm or up to 10,000 ppm. Many models of FIDs also have the configuration to work as a gas chromatograph, but this requires further training and experience to interpret the data correctly.

Gas Chromatographs

If a device such as a PID or FID does incorporate a gas chromatograph (GC), then the device can be set in one of two modes: first, only in the survey mode, which allows the device to run as a detector only, and second, in the GC mode, which allows the device to run as a detector and a GC. However, in this latter

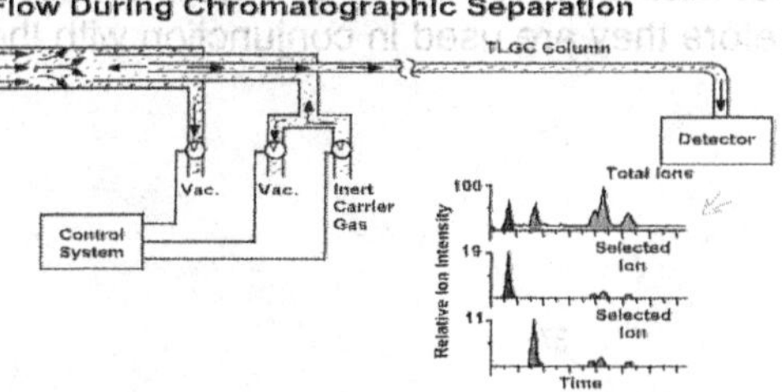

mode, proper use of the device requires extensive training and correct readings require near ideal conditions. In principle, a GC draws a test sample into a tube. The tube contains a medium that adsorbs the test sample with a variation in bonding strength. Depending on the strength of the bond, the sample is retained in the tube and eventually passed out the other end. This retention time is measured and compared to known relations of gases. Under ideal conditions of temperature, medium and flow rate, the GC can determine the quantity of a gas present based on retention time. It is possible to purchase a separate GC device for field use, but the cost (average $15,000) is a significant factor in most emergency response team's budget.

<u>Colorimetric Tubes</u>

The system that is used more often than PIDs and FIDs to determine unknown contaminants is colorimetric tubes. Although colorimetric tubes also have limitations and their use may be time consuming, they are far easier to use and maintain than PIDs and FIDs. Colorimetric tubes work on the principle of detecting a specific gas by having the test atmosphere drawn into a tube that is filled with a chemical that will change to a specific color in response to the gas.

Colorimetric tubes also can determine the quantity of gas present in parts per million. These markings, or n scale can be read to determine the level of contaminant based on the number of pump strokes required. However, any concentration reading should be taken as general due to slight variation in color, irregular changes in color, or a "bleeding" effect in color change. Thus the prime use of colorimetric tubes is to determine what actual gas is present but not its actual concentration. Colorimetric tube systems work well in identifying a specific gas, but results in actual levels in parts per million may vary from what is actually present by 25-50%. It is not necessary to purchase a tube for every type of contaminant. This would not only be extremely expensive, but also unwieldy. Manufacturers such as Drager and Sensidyne offer qualitative tubes for acids, bases, organic amines, unsaturated hydrocarbons, halogenated hydrocarbons, and aromatic hydrocarbons. Also offered are polytest tubes that detect multiple gases such as ammonia, hydrogen chloride, hydrogen sulfide, and chlorine.

Colorimetric tubes have some other considerations that may affect their use. Changes or extremes in temperature, high or low humidity, barometric pressure, sunlight, and other interfering gases may alter the reading. When taking readings, the user should always take three tubes: one to perform monitoring, the second to monitor if the first tube becomes saturated, and the third as a blank to determine subtle color changes. This assists in determining if there are any cross-sensitivities to the gas being measured. Each box of tubes has directions that describe any cross-sensitivities that may exist.

<u>Other Detection Devices</u>

Other monitors may be used in some situations to determine unknown contaminants in an atmosphere. As stated, if the presence of radioactive materials is known or suspected, then a device for measuring alpha, beta, and gamma radiation is used. There are also specialized monitors for materials such as lead, mercury, ozone, and solvent vapors that are used when a specific contaminant is suspected or known and verification is required.

Another type of air monitoring equipment that may sound rudimentary but can be essential is pH paper. If the presence of corrosive vapors is known or suspected, a simple procedure can protect sensitive equipment against corrosive vapors. Simply attach a piece of pH paper wetted with deionized water to an extension device as simple as a broom handle and put it into the test atmosphere. If the paper detects the presence of a strong corrosive gas (pH less than 2.5 or greater than 12), then ventilating the area or using some other engineering control can assist in reducing the level of contamination. Caution must be exercised even with an extension because you may still be contaminated by the atmosphere.

<u>General Procedures for Air Monitoring</u>

As with any piece of equipment, it is important to fully understand how it works before using it in the field. Becoming familiar with the monitor includes reading manufacturers' guidelines, practicing with other experienced personnel, and performing some basic drills before actual use. In addition, waste workers or responders shall be familiar with the procedures for calibrating and zeroing the monitor before use. Usually calibrating and zeroing requires energizing the monitor in a normal atmosphere before entering the test atmosphere. One of the prime reasons for equipment failure is not checking battery levels. Ensure all monitors to be used are properly charged and ready to go before use. Never go into the field with the faith that all equipment is in properly operating order. Involved personnel should know beforehand that all equipment is working properly. An ongoing maintenance program with a log that documents all work and tests performed is an excellent way to ensure air-monitoring equipment can be counted on when the need arises.

When testing for gases, it is important to remember that gases have different vapor densities. That is, some will rise and others will settle and possibly collect in low areas of the test atmosphere, therefore it is important to test high and low. Before entering a confined space, use an extension device to put the probe head of your oxygen meter or CGI into the space without making bodily entry. When using any sort of monitor, with or without an extension, allow time for the machine to draw the sample into the test chamber. The monitor pump may need a few moments before the sample reaches the detection device itself and is analyzed. In other words, do not keep walking into an area until you have a reading. Stop, wait a few moments, the proceed. Continue this process until the entire area has been tested. If dealing with a gas in a confined space or any enclosed area, think of the most logical place in which the gases may accumulate. Some gases stratify; they can occupy different layers dependent upon the vapor density of the associated atmosphere. Other gases such as hydrogen, acetylene, and ethylene may accumulate near the ceiling. Most hydrocarbon vapors and flammable gases such as propane and butane are heavier than air and lie low to the ground. These gases may follow the path of least resistance to the lowest area possible, therefore, it is important to check areas such as sumps, subfloors and trenches. When checking gases and vapors over liquid spills take care not to put a probe head into any standing liquid. Liquids, including water, that are drawn into the monitors, especially CGIs and PIDs, can alter readings and cause severe internal damage.

Monitoring In Confined Spaces

In confined spaces, it is important to remember that initial monitoring

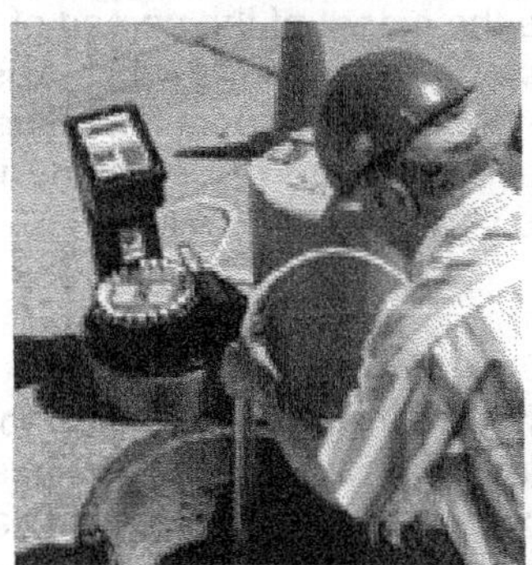

should be done without physical entry into the space. Attach extension devices to the probe head and wands if required. Keep in mind that any extension will increase the draw time. In the case of colorimetric tubes it may take the pump a long time to fully expand from each stroke. When monitoring confined spaces, ensure all corners are tested as well as any area that a suspect gas may pocket or accumulate. A good rule of thumb is that as much of the space as possible should be monitored. Monitoring in confined spaces, like all monitoring programs, shall continue as long as required; that is, several times during the workday, any time after workers have left the space and are returning, with any change in temperature or barometric pressure, if potential gases are produced or disturbed, or any other condition that may warrant monitoring the atmosphere. In many cases, monitors are kept energized from the beginning until the end of the task.

Monitoring Outside

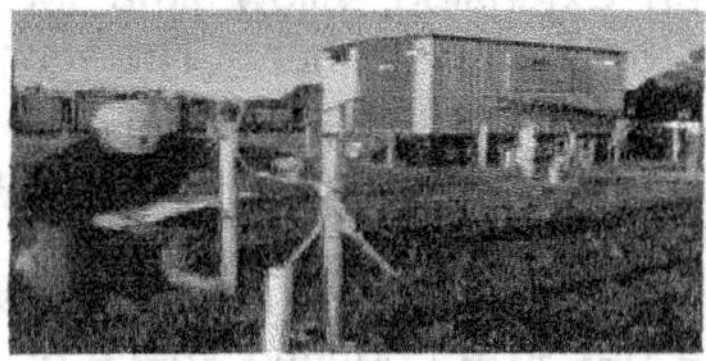

When monitoring outside, it is best to approach the spill from uphill and upwind if possible. Again, take a reasonable amount of time to allow the monitor to cycle what it is sampling. When outside, the use of an oxygen indicator is not usually required unless the gas discharge is large enough to displace the normal atmospheric oxygen level and is continuing to discharge. If a visible cloud is present and relatively stable conditions are in effect (no significant wind), then detection for oxygen deficiency may be required. It is a good idea to understand the effects of variations in topography. For example, heavy gases will follow the path of lease resistance into areas such a ravines, gullies, drainage ditches, and trenches. Remember too that many gases such as carbon monoxide are colorless and odorless and detection can be based only upon monitoring equipment.

Even after approaching from uphill and upwind, entry into the contamination area is necessary to detect what gas or vapor is present and the amount of contamination. Whenever this situation is encountered, proper personal protective equipment shall be used. Detection procedures shall include looking for a source or origin of the gas, such as a compromised cylinder, and then checking at various points downwind to determine the extent of the spread of the contamination. Monitoring should also be done on the cross-axis of the discharge area to determine the degree of dispersion. Finally, monitoring should be done upwind of the source to determine that there is no cross-contamination and to verify the source itself.

The Effects of Local Weather

Air monitoring procedures and the movement of gases and vapors can be significantly altered by changes in the weather. Changes in the temperature can increase vapor production (volatilization) and possibly lower vapor density, thus keeping gases near the ground instead of dissipating into the atmosphere. An increase in temperature may also affect the stability or reactivity of normally stable materials. With a change in temperature may also come a change in relative humidity. As the humidity level increases, so too may the rate of vaporization of water-based soluble material. The most significant weather event that may alter the situation is wind. In conditions of low wind (wind speed less than 10 knots), clouds of gases and vapors will be slow to dissipate and vapor concentration will remain high. When conditions are like this, the weather is considered stable and downwind dispersion remains small. When conditions become unstable (high winds and/or variation I wind direction), gas and vapors tend to spread further, but do disperse more rapidly. An increase in winds can also make dusts and particulate-bound contaminants airborne. With any task involving air monitoring, these factors should be taken into account along with planning for expected daily changes, called diurnal effects. Examples of diurnal effects are changes in barometric pressure, wind direction, and temperature.

When dealing with a release of a hazardous material it is very important to know the effects of local weather. In many situations outside agencies such as the National Weather Service or local airports can assist with weather forecasts. Land breezes and shore breezes to differences in the cooling ratios of land and water, wind tends to flow onshore or pick up velocity after about midday.

Because this effect can happen almost every day in some areas, it is a diurnal change that can be forecast with high accuracy. Thus, air monitoring would have to be continued to ensure contaminants are not being spread in a new or larger area due to any change in wind direction. If involved personnel desire more direct on-site weather readings, then more sophisticated equipment can be purchased. However, equipment required for weather monitoring does not have to be complex. A simple wind sock or any type of flag or banner waving from a pole can determine wind speed and direction.

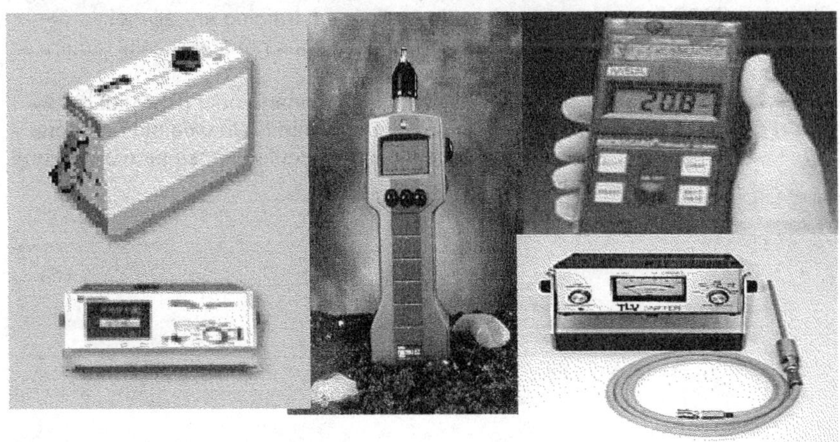

SUMMARY

- Emergency planning is a process of identifying hazards, analyzing risk, determining how to mitigate or reduce potential problems, developing response and recovery plans, developing procedures, conducting training, and then testing the plans with mock scenarios.
- The safety of employees and the public are the first priority in emergency planning and response.
- In general, a site plan is organized as a single document with the various component sections and appendixes covering all tasks, operations, and contractors/subcontractors or outsourced employees and can be used to promote efficiency and enhance completeness, clarity, and coordination.
- OSHA requires that all employers plan and prepare for emergencies in the workplace and that all employees be trained to perform whatever emergency response roles they are assigned.
- All employers, whether private or public are required to implement emergency action plans for emergencies in the workplace.
- The emergency action plan must include at least the following elements:
  1. Emergency escape procedures and emergency escape route assignments
  2. Procedures to be followed by employees who remain to operte critical site operations before evacuation (safe shut down)
  3. Procedures for accounting for employees after emergency evacuation is completed
  4. Rescue and medical assignments for designated employees
  5. Procedures for reporting fires and other emergencies
  6. Names and job titles of persons/departments who are responsible for the plan and can explain employee job duties under the plan.
- All employers must develop, implement, and maintain at each
- Workplace a written Hazard Communication Program that must include procedures to ensure that requirements for labels and other warnings, MSDAs, and employeee information and training are all met..
- The Hazard Communication Standard does not specifically require an emergency response plan.
- The major objective of process safety management (PSM) of highly hazardous chemicals is to prevent unwanted releases of hazardous chemicals, especially into locations that could expose employees and others to serious hazards.

Chapter 3 –TOXICOLOGY AND EXPOSURE GUIDELINES

"All substances are poisons; there is none which is not a poison. The right dose differentiates a poison and a remedy."

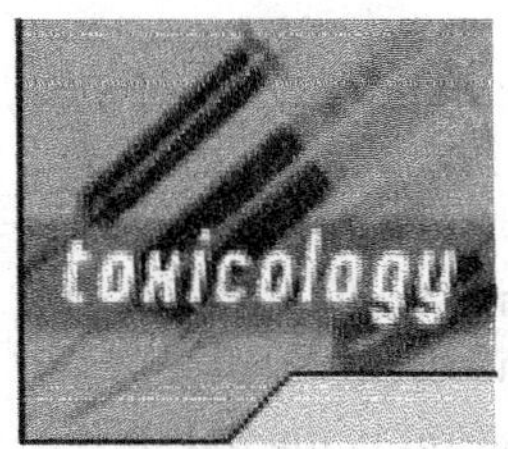

This early observation concerning the toxicity of chemicals was made by Paracelsus (1493-1541). The classic connotation of toxicology was "the science of poisons." Since that time, the science has expanded to encompass several disciplines. Toxicology is the study of the interaction between chemical agents and biological systems. While the subject of toxicology is quite complex, it is necessary to understand the basic concepts in order to make logical decisions concerning the protection of personnel from toxic injuries.

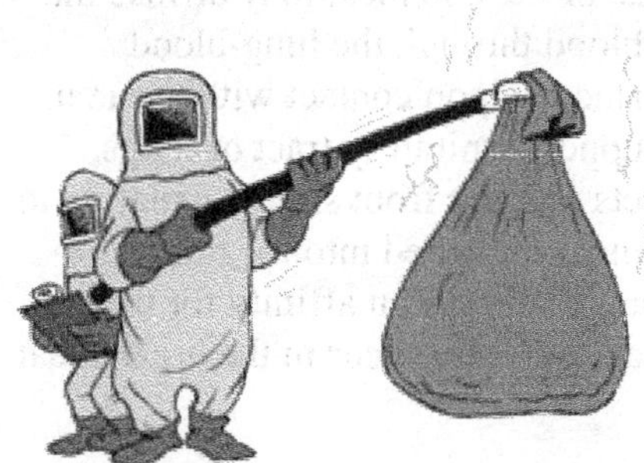

Toxicity can be defined as the relative ability of a substance to cause adverse effects in living organisms. This "relative ability" is dependent upon several conditions. As Paracelsus suggests, the quantity or the dose of the substance determines whether the effects of the chemical are toxic, non-toxic, or beneficial. In addition to dose, other factors may also influence the toxicity of the compound such as the route of entry, duration and frequency of exposure, variations between different species (interspecies), and variations among members of the same species (intraspecies).

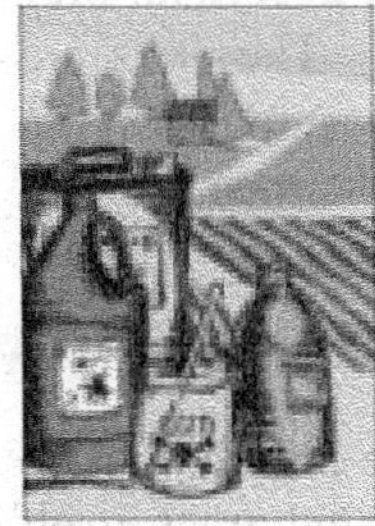

To apply these principles to hazardous materials response, the routes by which chemicals enter the human body will be considered first. Knowledge of these routes will support the selection of personal protective equipment and the development of safety plans. The second section deals with dose-response relationships. Since dose-response information is available in toxicology and chemistry reference books, it is useful to understand the relevance of these values to the concentrations that are actually measured in the environment. The third section of this chapter includes the effects of the duration and frequency of exposure, interspecies variation, and intraspecies variation on toxicity. Finally, toxic responses associated with chemical exposures are described according to each organ system.

Routes of Exposure

There are four routes by which a substance can enter the body: inhalation, skin (or eye) absorption, ingestion, and injection.

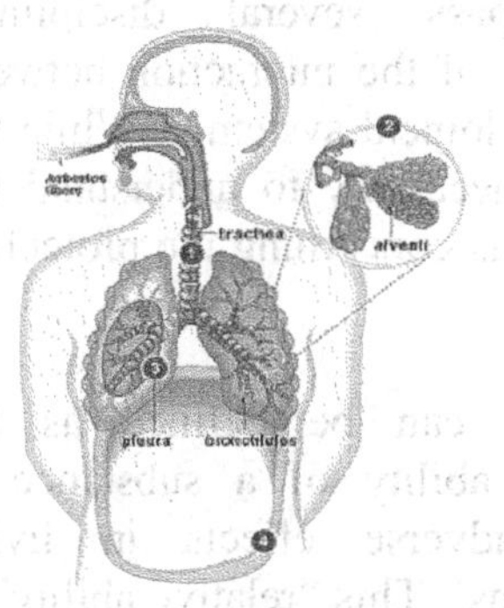

- **Inhalation**: For most chemicals in the form of vapors, gases, mists, or particulates, inhalation is the major route of entry. Once inhaled, chemicals are either exhaled or deposited in the respiratory tract. If deposited, damage can occur through direct contact with tissue or the chemical may diffuse into the blood through the lung-blood interface. Upon contact with tissue in the upper respiratory tract or lungs, chemicals may cause health effects ranging from simple irritation to severe tissue destruction. Substances absorbed into the blood are circulated and distributed to organs that have an affinity for that particular chemical. Health effects can then occur in the organs that are sensitive to the toxicant.

- **Skin (or eye) absorption**: Skin (dermal) contact can cause effects that are relatively innocuous such as redness or mild dermatitis; more severe effects include destruction of skin tissue or other debilitating conditions. Many chemicals can also cross the skin barrier and be absorbed into the blood system. Once absorbed, they may produce systemic damage to internal organs. The eyes are particularly sensitive to chemicals. Even a short exposure can cause severe effects to the eyes or the substance can be absorbed through the eyes and be transported to other parts of the body causing harmful effects.

- **Ingestion**: Chemicals that inadvertently get into the mouth and are swallowed do not generally harm the gastrointestinal tract itself unless they are irritating or corrosive. Chemicals that are insoluble in the fluids of the gastrointestinal tract (stomach, small, and large intestines) are generally excreted. Others that are soluble are absorbed through the lining of the gastrointestinal tract. They are then transported by the blood to internal organs, where they can cause damage.

- **Injection**: Substances may enter the body if the skin is penetrated or punctured by contaminated objects. Effects can then occur as the substance is circulated in the blood and deposited in the target organs.

Once the chemical is absorbed into the body, three other processes are possible: metabolism, storage, and excretion. Many chemicals are metabolized or transformed via chemical reactions in the body. In come cases, chemicals are distributed and stored in specific organs. Storage may reduce metabolism and therefore, increase the persistence of the chemicals in the body. The various excretory mechanisms (exhaled breath, perspiration, urine, feces, or detoxification) rid the body, over a period of time, of the chemical. For some chemicals, elimination may be a matter of days or months; for others, the elimination rate is so low that they may persist in the body for a lifetime and cause deleterious effects.

The Dose-Response Relationship

In general, a given amount of a toxic agent will elicit a given type and intensity of response. The dose-response relationship is a fundamental concept in toxicology and the basis for measurement of the relative harmfulness of a chemical. A dose-response relationship is defined as a consistent mathematical and biologically plausible correlation between the number of individuals responding and a given dose over an exposure period.

Dose Terms. In toxicology, studies of the dose given to test organisms is expressed in terms of the quantity administered:

- **Quantity per unit mass (or weight).** Usually expressed as milligram per kilogram of body weight (mg/kg).

- **Quantity per unit area of skin surface.** Usually expressed as milligram per square centimeter (mg/cm^2).

- **Volume of substance in air per unit volume of air.** Usually given as microliters of vapor or gas per liter of air by volume (ppm). Particulates and gases are also given as milligrams of material per cubic meter of air (mg/m^3).

The period of time over which a dose has been administered is generally specified. For example, 5 mg/kg/3 D is 5 milligrams of chemical per kilogram of the subject's body weight administered over a period of three days. For dose to be meaningful, it must be related to the effect it causes. For example, 50 mg/kg of chemical "X" administered orally to female rats has no relevancy unless the effect of the dose, say sterility in all test subjects, is reported.

Dose-Response Curves. A dose-response relationship is represented by a dose-response curve. The curve is generated by plotting the dose of the chemical versus the response in the test population. There are a number of ways to present this data. One of the more common methods for presenting the dose-response curve is shown in **GRAPH 1**. In this example, the dose is expressed in "mg/kg" and depicted on the "x" axis. The response is expressed as a "cumulative percentage" of animals in the test population that exhibit the specific health effect under study. Values for "cumulative percentage" are indicated on the "y" axis of the graph. As the dose increases, the percentage of the affected population increases.

Dose-response curves provide valuable information regarding the potency of the compound. The curves are also used to determine the dose-response terms that are discussed in the following section.

GRAPH 1
HYPOTHETICAL DOSE-RESPONSE CURVE

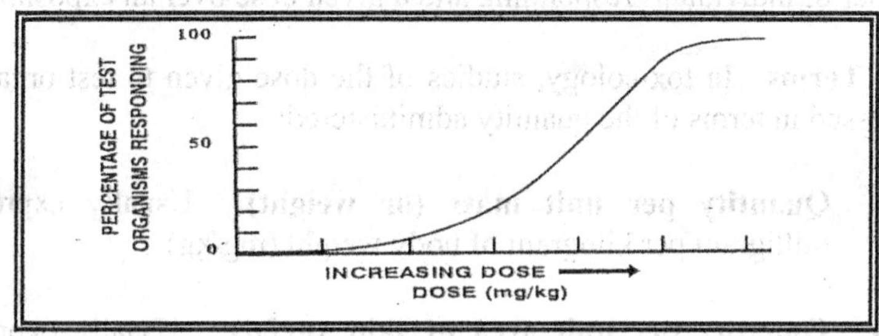

Dose-Response Terms. The National Institute for Occupational Safety and Health (NIOSH) defines a number of general dose-response terms in the "Registry of Toxic Substances" A summary of these terms is contained in **TABLE 1**.

- **Toxic dose low (TD_{LO})**: The lowest dose of a substance introduced by any route, other than inhalation, over any given period of time, and reported to produce any toxic effect in humans or to produce tumorigenic or reproductive effects in animals.

- **Toxic concentration low (TC_{LO})**: The lowest concentration of a substance in air to which humans or animals have been exposed for any given period of time that has produced any toxic effect in humans or produced tumorigenic or reproductive effects in animals.

- **Lethal dose low (LD_{LO})**: The lowest dose, other than LD_{50}, of a substance introduced by any route, other than inhalation, which has been reported to have caused death in humans or animals.

- **Lethal dose fifty (LD_{50})**: A calculated dose of a substance which is expected to cause the death of 50 percent of an entire defined experimental animal population. It is determined from the exposure to the substance by any route other than inhalation.

- **Lethal concentration low (LC_{LO})**: The lowest concentration of a substance in air, other than LC_{50}, which has been reported to have caused death in humans or animals.

- **Lethal concentration fifty (LC_{50})**: A calculated concentration of a substance in air, exposure to which for a specified length of time is expected to cause the death of 50 percent of an entire defined experimental animal population.

Limitations of Dose-Response Terms. Several limitations must be recognized when using dose-response data. First, it is difficult to select a test species that will closely duplicate the human response to a specific chemical. For example, human data indicates that arsenic is a carcinogen, while animal studies do not demonstrate these results. Second, most lethal and toxic dose data are derived from acute (single dose, short-term) exposures rather than chronic (continuous, long-term) exposures. A third shortcoming is that the LD_{50} or LC_{50} is a single value and does not indicate the toxic effects that may occur at different dose levels. For example, in **GRAPH 2**, Chemical A is assumed to be more toxic than Chemical B based on Ld$_{50}$, but at lower doses the situation is reversed. At LD$_{20}$, Chemical B is more toxic than Chemical A.

TABLE 1
SUMMARY OF DOSE-RESPONSE TERMS

Category	Exposure Time	Route of Exposure	Toxic Effects Human	Toxic Effects Animal
TD$_{LO}$	Acute or chronic	All except inhalation	Any non-lethal	Reproductive, Tumorigenic
TC$_{LO}$	Acute or chronic	Inhalation	Any non-lethal	Reproductive, Tumorigenic
LD$_{LO}$	Acute or chronic	All except inhalation	Death	Death
LD$_{50}$	Acute	All except inhalation	Not applicable	Death (statistically determined)
LC$_{LO}$	Acute or chronic	Inhalation	Death	Death
LC$_{50}$	Acute	Inhalation	Not applicable	Death (statistically determined)

GRAPH 2
COMPARISON OF DOSE-RESPONSE CURVES FOR TWO SUBSTANCES

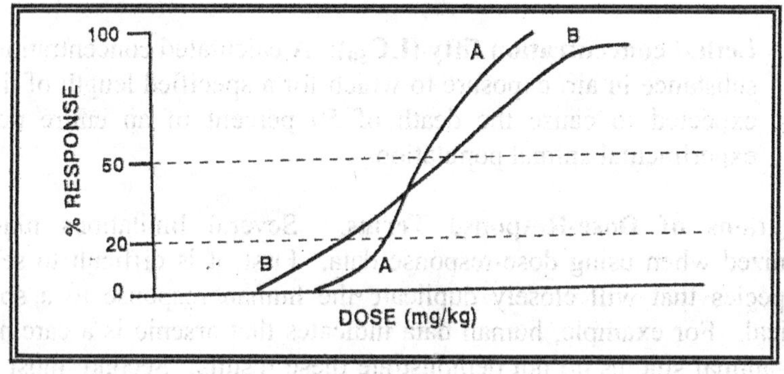

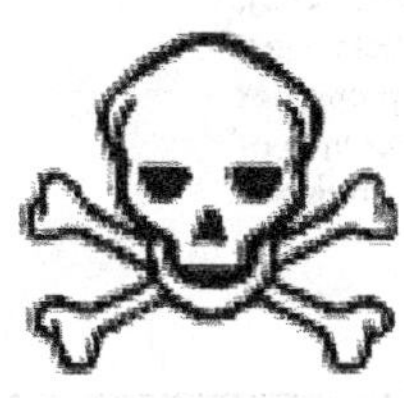

Factors Influencing Toxicity. Many factors affect the reaction of an organism to a toxic chemical. The specific response that is elicited by a given dose varies depending on the species being tested and variations that occur among individuals of the same species. These must be considered when using information such as that found in **TABLE 2**.

- **Duration and Frequency of Exposure**. There is a difference in type and severity of effects depending on how rapidly the dose is received (duration) and how often the dose is received (frequency). Acute exposures are usually single incidents of relatively short duration – a minute to a few days. Chronic exposures involve frequent doses at relatively low levels over a period of time ranging from months to years.

  If a dose is administered slowly so that the rate of elimination or the rate of detoxification keeps pace with intake, it is possible that no toxic response will occur. The same dose could produce an effect with rapid administration.

TABLE 2
CLASSIFICATION OF FACTORS INFLUENCING TOXICITY

TYPE	EXAMPLES
Factors related to the chemical	Composition (salt, free base, etc.); physical characteristics (particle size, liquid, solid, etc.); physical properties (volatility, solubility, etc.); presence of impurities; break down products; carrier
Factors related to exposure	Dose; concentration; route of exposure (ingestion, skin absorption, injection, inhalation); duration.
Factors related to person exposed	Heredity; immunology; nutrition; hormones; age; sex; health status; pre-existing disease.
Factors related to environment	Carrier (air, water, food, soil); additional chemical present (synergism, antagonism); temperature; air pressure.

- **Routes of Exposure**. Biological results can be different for the same dose, depending on whether the chemical is inhaled, ingested, applied to the skin, or injected. Natural barriers impede the intake and distribution of material once in the body. These barriers can accenuate the toxic effects of the same dose of a chemical. The effectiveness of these barriers is partially dependent upon the route of entry of the chemical.

- **Interspecies Variation**. For the same dose received under identical conditions, the effects exhibited by different species may vary greatly. A dose that is lethal for one species may have no effect on another. Since the toxicological effects of chemicals on humans is usually based on animal studies, a test species must be selected that most closely approximates the physiological processes of humans.

- **Intraspecies Variations**. Within a given species, not all members of the population respond to the same dose identically. Some members will be more sensitive to the chemical and elicit response at lower doses than the more resistant members that require larger doses for the same response.

- Age and Maturity. Infants and children are often more sensitive to toxic action than younger adults. Elderly persons have diminished physiological capabilities for the body to deal with toxic insult. These age groups may be more susceptible to toxic effects at relatively lower doses.

- Gender and Hormonal Status. Some chemicals may be more toxic to one gender than the other. Certain chemicals can affect the reproductive system of either the male or female. Additionally, since women have a larger percentage of body fat than men, they may accumulate more fat-soluble chemicals. Some variations in response have also been shown to be related to physiological differences between males and females.

- Genetic Makeup. Genetic factors influence individual responses to toxic substances. If the necessary physiological processes are diminished or defective, the natural body defenses are impaired. For example, people lacking in the G6PD enzyme (a hereditary abnormality) are more likely to suffer red blood cell damage when given aspirin or certain antibiotics than persons with the normal form of the enzyme.

- State of Health. Persons with poor health are generally more susceptible to toxic damage due to the body's decreased capability to deal with chemical insult.

- **Environmental Factors**. Environmental factors may contribute to the response for a given chemical. For example, such factors as air pollution, workplace conditions, living conditions, personal habits, and previous chemical exposure may act in conjunction with other toxic mechanisms.

- **Chemical Combinations**. Some combinations of chemicals produce different effects from those attributed to each individually:

- Synergists: chemicals that, when combined, cause a greater than additive effect. For example, hepatotoxicity is enhanced as a result of exposure to both ethanol and carbon tetrachloride.
- Potentiation: is a type of synergism where the potentiator is not usually toxic in itself, but has the ability to increase the toxicity of other chemicals. Isopropanol, for example, is not hepatotoxic in itself. Its combination with carbon tetrachloride, however, increases the toxic response to the carbon tetrachloride.
- Antagonists: chemicals, that when combined, lessen the predicted effect. There are four types of antagonists.

(1) functional: Produces opposite effects on the same physiologic function. For example, phosphate reduces lead absorption in the gastrointestinal tract by forming insoluble lead phosphate.

(2) chemical: Reacts with the toxic compound to form a less toxic product. For example, chelating agents bind up metals such as lead, arsenic, and mercury.

(3) dispositional: Alters absorption, metabolism, distribution, or excretion. For example, some alcohols use the same enzymes in their metabolism:

$$\text{ethanol} \longrightarrow \text{acetaldehyde} \longrightarrow \text{acetic acid}$$
$$\text{methanol} \longrightarrow \text{formaldehyde} \longrightarrow \text{formic acid}$$

The aldehydes cause toxic effects (hangover, blindness). Ethanol is more readily metabolized than methanol, so when both are present, methanol is not metabolized and can be excreted before forming formaldehyde. Another dispositional antagonist is Antabuse which, when administered to alcoholics, inhibits the metabolism of acetaldehyde, giving the patient a more severe prolonged hangover.

(4) receptor: Occurs when a second chemical either binds to the same tissue receptor as a toxic chemical or blocks the

action of receptor and thereby reduces the toxic effect. For example, atropine interferes with the receptor responsible for the toxic effects of organophosphate pesticides.

Sources of Toxicity Information

Information on the toxic properties of chemical compounds and dose-response relationships is obtained from animal studies, epidemiological investigations of exposed human populations, and clinical studies or case reports of exposed humans.

- **Toxicity Tests.** The design of any toxicity test incorporates:

    - a test organism, which can range from cellular material and selected strains of bacteria through higher order plants and animals
    - a response or biological endpoint, which can range from subtle changes in physiology and behavior to death
    - an exposure or test period
    - a dose or series of doses

    The objective is to select a test species that is a good model of humans, a response that is not subjective and can be consistently determined for a given dose, and a test period that is relatively short.

- **Epidemiological and Clinical Studies.** Epidemiological investigations and clinical cases are another means of relating human health effects and exposure to toxic substances. Epidemiological investigations are based upon a human population exposed to a chemical compared to an appropriate, non-exposed group. An attempt is made to determine whether there is a statistically significant association between health effects and chemical exposure. Clinical cases involve individual reports of chemical exposure.

Uses of Toxicity Information

Comparison of Toxicity Data. Comparing the LD_{50} of chemicals in animals gives a relative ranking of potency or toxicity of each. For example, DDT (LD_{50} for rats = 14,000 mg/kg). Using the LD_{50} (mg/kg) for a test species and multiplying by 70 kg (average mass of man) gives a rough estimate of the toxic potential of the substance for humans, assuming that humans are as sensitive as the subjects tested.

Since the extrapolation of human data from animal studies is complex, this value should only be considered as an approximation for the potency of the compound and used in conjunction with additional data (**TABLES 3 and 4**).

Establishing Exposure Guidelines. Toxicity data from both animal experimentation and epidemiological studies is used to establish exposure guidelines. The method for deriving a guideline is dependent upon the type of chemical as well as duration and frequency of exposure. It is also important to make the distinction between an experimental dose (mg/kg) and an environmental concentration (mg/m^3 or ppm). In order to make safety decisions, exposure guidelines are presented as concentrations so that these values can be compared to concentrations measured by air monitoring instrumentation.

TABLE 3	
TOXICITY RATING TABLE	
Toxicity Rating or Class	Oral Acute LD 50 for RATS
Extremely toxic	1 mg/kg or less (dioxin, botulinum toxin)
Highly toxic	
	1 to 50 mg/kg (strychnine)
Moderately toxic	
	50 to 500 mg/kg (DDT)
Slightly toxic	
	0.5 to 5 g/kg (morphine)
Practically nontoxic	
	5 to 15 g/kg (ethyl alcohol

TABLE 4
TABLE OF LD50 VALUES FOR RATS FOR A
GROUP OF WELL-KNOWN CHEMICALS

Chemical	LD50 (mg/kg)
	29,700
Sucrose (table sugar)	14,000
Ethyl alcohol	3,000
Sodium chloride (common	2,000
salt)	1,580
Vitamin A	1,000
Vanillin	800
Aspirin	300
Chloroform	192
Copper sulfate	162
Caffeine	113
Phenobarbital, sodium salt	85
DDT	53
Sodium nitrite	7
Nicotine	6.4
Aflatoxin B1	2.5
Sodium cyanide	
Strychnine	

Health Effects

Human health effects caused by exposure to toxic substances fall into two
categories: short-term and long-term effects. Short-term effects (or **acute
effects**) have a relatively quick onset (usually minutes to days) after brief
exposures to relatively high concentrations of material (acute exposures).
The effect may be local or systemic. Local effects occur at the site of
contact between the toxicant and the body. This site is usually the skin or
eyes, but includes the lungs if irritants are inhaled, or the gastrointestinal
tract if corrosives are ingested. Systemic effects are those that occur if the
toxicant has been absorbed into the body from its initial contact point,
transported to other parts of the body, and cause adverse effects in
susceptible organs. Many chemicals can cause both local and systemic
effects.

Long-term effects (or **chronic effects**) are those with a long period of time (years) between exposure and injury. These effects may occur after apparent recovery from acute exposure or as a result of repeated exposures to low concentrations of materials over a period of years (chronic exposure).

Health effects manifested from acute or chronic exposure are dependent upon the chemical involved and the organ it affects. Most chemicals do not exhibit the same degree of toxicity for all organs.

Usually the major effects of a chemical will be expressed in one or two organs. These organs are known as target organs, which are more sensitive to that particular chemical than other organs. The organs of the body and examples of effects due to chemical exposures are listed below.

Respiratory Tract. The respiratory tract is the only organ system with vital functional elements in constant, direct contact with the environment. The lung also has the largest exposed surface area of any organ on a surface area of 70 to 100 square meters versus two square meters for the skin and 10 square meters for the digestive system.

The respiratory tract is divided into three regions: (1) Nasopharyngeal – extends from nose to larynx. These passages are lined with ciliated epithelium and mucous glands. They filter out large inhaled particles, increase the relative humidity of inhaled air, and moderate its temperature. (2) Tracheobronchial – consists of trachea, bronchi, and bronchioles and serves as conducting airway epithelium coated by mucous, which serves as an escalator to move particles from deep in the lungs back up to the oral cavity so they can be swallowed. These ciliated cells can be temporarily paralyzed by smoking or using cough suppressants. (3) Pulmonary acinus – is the basic functional unit in the lung and the primary location of gas exchange. It consists of small bronchioles that connect to the alveoli. The alveoli, of which there are 100 million in humans, contact the pulmonary capillaries.

Inhaled particles settle in the respiratory tract according to their diameters:

- 5-30 micron are deposited in the nasopharyngeal region.
- 1-5 micron are deposited in the tracheobronchial region.
- Less than 1 micron are deposited in the alveolar region by diffusion and Brownian motion.

In general, most particles 5-10 microns in diameter are removed. However, certain small inorganic particles, settle into smaller regions of the lung and kill the cells that attempt to remove them. The result is fibrous lesions of the lung.

Many chemicals used or produced in industry can produce acute or chronic diseases of the respiratory tract when they are inhaled (**TABLE 5**). The toxicants can be classified according to how they affect the respiratory tract.

- **Asphyxiants**: gases that deprive the body tissues of oxygen.
- **Simple asphyxiants** are physiologically inert gases that at high concentrations displace air leading to suffocation. Examples: nitrogen, helium, methane, neon, argon.
- **Chemical asphyxiants** are gases that prevent the tissues from getting enough oxygen. Examples: carbon monoxide and cyanide. Carbon monoxide binds to hemoglobin 200 times more readily than oxygen. Cyanide prevents the transfer of oxygen from blood to tissues by inhibiting the necessary transfer enzymes.
- **Irritants**: chemicals that irritate the air passages. Constriction of the airways occurs and may lead to edema (liquid in the lungs) and infection. Examples: hydrogen fluoride, chlorine, hydrogen chloride, and ammonia.
- **Necrosis producers**: Chemicals that result in cell death and edema. Examples: ozone and nitrogen dioxide.
- **Fibrosis producers**: Chemicals that produce fibrotic tissue which, if massive, blocks airways and decreases lung capacity. Examples: silicates, asbestos, and beryllium
- **Allergens**: Chemicals that induce an allergic response characterized by bronchoconstriction and pulmonary disease. Examples: isocyanates and sulfur dioxide.
- **Carcinogens**: Chemicals that are associated with lung cancer. Examples: cigarette smoke, coke oven emissions, asbestos, and arsenic.

Not only can various chemicals affect the respiratory tract, but the tract is also a route for chemicals to reach other organs. Solvents, such as benzene and tetrachloroethane, anesthetic gases, and many other chemical compounds can be absorbed through the respiratory tract and cause systemic effects.

TABLE 5
EXAMPLES OF INDUSTRIAL TOXICANTS THAT PRODUCE
DISEASE OF THE RESPIRATORY TRACT

TOXICANT	SITE OF ACTION	ACUTE EFFECT	CHRONIC EFFECT
Ammonia	Upper airways	Irritation, edema	Bronchitis
Arsenic	Upper airways	Bronchitis, irritation, pharyngitis	Cancer, bronchitis, laryngitis
Asbestos	Lung parenchyma	- - - - - - - - - -	Fibrosis, cancer
Chlorine	Upper airways	Cough, irritation, asphyxiant (by muscle cramps in larynx)	- - - - - - - - - -
Isocyanates	Lower airways, alveoli	Bronchitis, pulmonary edema, asthma	- - - - - - - - - -
Nickel Carbony	Alveoli	Edema (delayed symptoms)	- - - - - - - - - -
Ozone	Bronchi, alveoli	Irritation, edema, hemorrhage	Emphysema, bronchitis
Phosgene	Alveoli	Edema	Bronchitis, fibrosis, pneumonia
Toluene	Upper airways	Bronchitis, edema, bronchospasm	- - - - - - - - - -
Xylene	Lower airways	Edema, hemorrhage	- - - - - - - - - -

Skin. The skin is, in terms of weight, the largest single organ of the body. It provides a barrier between the environment and other organs (except the lungs and eyes) and is a defense against many chemicals.

The skin consists of the epidermis (outer layer) and the dermis (inner layer). In the dermis are sweat glands and ducts, sebaceous glands, connective tissue, fat, hair follicles, and blood vessels. Hair follicles and sweat glands penetrate both the epidermis and dermis. Chemicals can penetrate through the sweat glands, sebaceous glands, or hair follicles.

Although the follicles and glands may permit a small amount of chemicals to enter almost immediately, most pass through the epidermis, which constitutes the major surface area. The top layer is the stratum corneum, a thin cohesive membrane of dead surface skin. This layer turns over every two weeks by a complex process of cell dehydration and polymerization of intracellular material. The epidermis plays the critical role in skin permeability.

Below the epidermis lies the dermis, a collection of cells providing a porous, watery, nonselective diffusion medium. Intact skin has a number of functions:

- Epidermis: Prevents absorption of chemicals and is a physical barrier to bacteria.
- Sebaceous glands: Secrete fatty acids which are bacteriostatic and fungistatic.
- Melanocytes (skin pigment): Prevent damage from ultraviolet radiation in sunlight.
- Sweat glands: Regulate heat.
- Connective tissue: Provides elasticity against trauma.
- Lymph-blood system: Provide immunologic responses to infection.

The ability of skin to absorb foreign substances depends on the properties and health of the skin and the chemical properties of the substances. Absorption is enhanced by:

- Breaking top layer of skin by abrasions or cuts.
- Increasing hydration of skin.
- Increasing temperature of skin which causes sweat cells to open up and secrete sweat, which can dissolve solids.
- Increasing blood flow to skin.
- Increasing concentrations of the substance.
- Increasing contact time of the chemical on the skin.
- Increasing the surface area of affected skin.
- Altering the skin's normal pH of 5.
- Decreasing particle size of substance.
- Adding agents that will damage skin and render it more susceptible to penetration.

- Adding surface-active agents or organic chemicals. DMSO, for example, can act as a carrier of the substance.
- Inducing ion movement by an electrical charge.

Absorption of a toxic chemical through the skin can lead to: **local effects**, such as irritation and necrosis, through direct contact and **systemic effects**.

Many chemicals can cause a reaction with the skin resulting in inflammation called dermatitis. These chemicals are divided into three categories:

- **Primary irritants**: Act directly on normal skin at the site of contact (if chemical is in sufficient quantity for a sufficient length of time). Skin irritants include: acetone, benzyl chloride, carbon disulfide, chloroform, chromic acid and other soluble chromium compounds, ethylene oxide, hydrogen chloride, iodine, methyl ethyl ketone, mercury, phenol, phosgene, styrene, sulfur dioxide, picric acid, toluene, xylene.

- **Photosensitizers**: Increase in sensitivity to light, which results in irritation and redness. Photosensitizers include: tetracyclines, acridine, creosote, pyridine, furfural, and naphtha.

- **Allergic sensitizers**: May produce allergic-type reaction after repeated exposures. They include: formaldehyde, phthalic anhydride, ammonia, mercury, nitrobenzene, toluene diisocyanate, chromic acid and chromates, cobalt, and benzoyl peroxide.

Eyes. The eyes are affected by the same chemicals that affect skin, but the eyes are much more sensitive. Many materials can damage the eyes by direct contact:

- **Acids**: Damage to the eye by acids depends on pH and the protein-combining capacity of the acid. Unlike alkali burns, the acid burns that are apparent during the first few hours are a good indicator of the long-term damage to be expected. Some acids and their properties are:

    - sulfuric acid. In addition to its acid properties, it simultaneously removes water and generates heat.
    - picric acid and tannic acid. No difference in damage they produce in entire range of acidic pHs.

- hydrochloric acid. Severe damage at pH 1, but no effect at pH 3 or greater.

- **Alkalies**: Damage that appears mild initially but can later lead to ulceration, perforation, and clouding of the cornea or lens. The pH and length of exposure have more bearing on the amount of damage than the type of alkali. Some problem alkalies are:

  - sodium hydroxide (caustic soda) and potassium hydroxide.
  - Ammonia penetrates eye tissues more readily than any other alkali; calcium oxide (lime) forms clumps when it contacts eye tissue and is very hard to remove.

- **Organic solvents**: Organic solvents (for example, ethanol, toluene, and acetone) dissolve fats, cause pain, and dull the cornea. Damage is usually slight unless the solvent is hot.

- **Lacrimators**: Lacrimators cause instant tearing at low concentrations. They are distinguished from other eye irritants (hydrogen chloride and ammonia) because they induce an instant reaction without damaging tissues. At very high concentrations lacrimators can cause chemical burns and destroy corneal material. Examples are chloroacetophenone (tear gas) and mace.

In addition, some compounds act on eye tissue to form cataracts, damage the optic nerve, or damage the retina. These compounds usually reach the eye through the blood system having been inhaled, ingested, or absorbed rather than direct contact.

Examples of compounds that can provide systemic effects damaging to the eyes are:

  - Naphthalene: Cataracts and retina damage.
  - Phenothiazine (insecticide): Retina damage.
  - Thallium: cataracts and optic nerve damage.
  - Methanol: Optic nerve damage.

Central Nervous System. Neurons (nerve cells) have a high metabolic rate but little capacity for anaerobic metabolism. Subsequently, inadequate oxygen flow (anoxia) to the brain kills cells within minutes. Some may die before oxygen or glucose transport stops completely.

Because of their need for oxygen, nerve cells are readily affect by both simple asphyxiants and chemical asphyxiants. Also, their ability to receive adequate oxygen is affected by compounds that reduce respiration and thus reduce oxygen content of the blood (barbiturates, narcotics). Other examples are compounds such as arsine, nickel, ethylene chlorohydrin, tetraethyl lead, aniline, and benzene that reduce blood pressure or flow due to cardiac arrest, extreme hypotension, hemorrhaging, or thrombosis.

Some compounds damage neurons or inhibit their function through specific action on parts of the cell. The major symptoms from such damage include: dullness, restlessness, muscle tremor, convulsions, loss of memory, epilepsy, idiocy, loss of muscle coordination, and abnormal sensations. Examples are:

- Fluoroacetate: Rodenticide.
- Triethyltin: Ingredient of insectcides and fungicides.
- Hexachlorophene: Antibacterial agent.
- Lead: Gasoline additive and paint ingredient.
- Thallium: Sulfate used as a pesticide and oxide or carbonate used in manufacture of optical glass and artificial gems.
- Tellurium: Pigment in glass and porcelain.
- Organomercury compounds: Methyl mercury used as a fungicide; is also a product of microbial action on mercury ions. Organomercury compounds are especially hazardous because of their volatility and their ability to permeate tissue barriers.

Some chemicals are noted for producing weakness of the lower extremities and abnormal sensations (along with previously mentioned symptoms):

- Acrylamide: Soil stabilizer, waterproofer.
- Carbon disulfide: Solvent in rayon and rubber industries.
- N-Hexane: Used as a cleaning fluid and solvent. Its metabolic product, hexanedione, causes the effects.
- Organophosphorus compounds: Often used as flame retardants (triorthocresyl phosphate) and pesticides (Leptofor and Mipafox).

Agents that prevent the nerves from producing proper muscle contraction and may result in death from respiratory paralysis are DDT, lead, botulinum toxin, and allethrin (a synthetic insecticide). DDT, mercury, manganese; and monosodium glutamate also produce personality disorders and madness.

Liver. Liver injury induced by chemicals has been known as a toxicologic problem for hundreds of years. It was recognized early that liver injury is not a simple entity, but that the type of lesion depends on the chemical and duration of exposure. Three types of response to hepatotoxins can be identified:

- **Acute**. Cell death from:

    - carbon tetrachloride: Solvent, degreaser.
    - chloroform: Used in refrigerant manufacture solvent.
    - trichloroethylene: Solvent, dry cleaning fluid, degreaser.
    - tetrachloroethane: Paint and varnish remover, dry cleaning fluid.
    - bromobenzene: Solvent, motor oil additive.
    - tannic acid: Ink manufacture, beer and wine clarifier.
    - kepone: Pesticide.1

- **Chronic**. Examples include:

    - cirrhosis: a progressive fibrotic disease of the liver associated with liver dysfunction and jaundice. Among agents implicated in cirrhosis cases are carbon tetrachloride, alcohol, and aflatoxin.
    - carcinomas: malignant, growing tissue. For example, vinyl chloride (used in polyvinyl chloride production) and arsenic (used in pesticides and paints) are associated with cancers.

- **Biotransformation of toxicants**. The liver is the principal organ that chemically alters all compounds entering the body. For example:

    ethanol--- >acetaldehyde---> acetic acid-> water + carbon dioxide

This metabolic action by the liver can be affected by diet, hormone activity, and alcohol consumption. Biotransformation in the liver can also lead to toxic metabolities. For example:

carbon tetrachloride---> chloroform

Kidneys. The kidney is susceptible to toxic agents for several reasons: (1) The kidneys constitute one percent of the body's weight, but receive 20-25 percent of the blood flow (during rest). Thus, large amounts of circulating toxicants reach the kidneys quickly. (2 The kidneys have high oxygen and nutrient requirements because of their work load. They filter 1/3 of the plasma reaching them and reabsorb 98-99% of the salt and water. As they are reabsorbed, salt concentrates in the kidneys. (3) Changes in kidney pPH may increase passive diffusion and thus cellular concentrations of toxicants. (4) Active secretion processes may concentrate toxicants. (5) Biotransformation is high.

A number of materials are toxic to the kidneys.

- Heavy metals may denature proteins as well as produce cell toxicity. Heavy metals (including mercury, chromium, arsenic, gold, cadmium, lead, and silver) are readily concentrated in the kidneys, making this organ particularly sensitive.

- Halogenated organic compounds, which contain chlorine, fluorine, bromine, or iodine. Metabolism of these compounds, like that occurring in the liver, generates toxic metabolites. Among compounds toxic to the kidneys are carbon tetrachloride, chloroform, 2,4,5-T (a herbicide), and ethylene dibroamide (a fumigant).

- Miscellaneous, including carbon disulfide (solvent for waxes and resinsa) and ethlene glycol (automobile antifreeze).

Blood. The blood system can be damaged by agents that affect blood cell production (bone marrow), the components of blood (platelets, red blood cells, and white blood cells), or the oxygen-carrying capacity of red blood cells.

Bone Marrow. Bone marrow is the source of most components in the blood. Agents that suppress the function of bone marrow include:

- Arsenic, used in pesticides and paints.
- Bromine, used to manufacture gasoline antiknock compounds, ethylene dibromide, and organic dyes.
- Methyl chloride, used as a solvent, refrigerant, and aerosol propellant.
- Ionizing radiation, produced by radioactive materials and x-rays is associated with leukemia.
- Benzine, a chemical intermediate associated with leukemia.

Blood Components. Among platelets (thrombocytes) are blood components that help prevent blood loss by forming blood clots. Among chemicals that affect this action are:

- Aspirin, which inhibits clotting.
- Benzene, which decreases the number of platelets.
- Tetrachloroethane, which increases the number of platelets.

Leukocytes (white blood cells) are primarily responsible for defending the body against foreign organisms or materials by engulfing and destroying the material or by producing antibodies. Chemicals that increase the number of leukocytes include naphthalene, magnesium oxide, boron hydrides, and tetrachloroethane. Agents that decrease the number of leukocytes include benzene and phosphorous.

Erthrocytes (red blood cells) transport oxygen in the blood. Chemicals that destroy (hemolyze) red blood cells include arsine (a gaseous arsenic compound and contaminant in acetylene), naphthalene (used to make dyes), and warfarin (a rodenticide).

Oxygen Transport. Some compounds affect the oxygen carrying capabilities of red blood cells. A notable example is carbon monoxide, which combines with hemoglobin to form carboxyhemoglovin. Hemoglobin has an affinity for carbon monoxide 200 times greater than that for oxygen.

While carbon monoxide combines reversibly with hemoglobin, some chemicals cause the hemoglobin to change such that it cannot combine reversibly with oxygen. This condition is called methemoglobinemia. Some chemicals that can cause this are:

- Sodium nitrite, used in meat curing and photography.
- Aniline, used in manufacture of rubber accelerators and antioxidants, resins, and varnishes.
- Nitrobenzene and dinitrobenzene, used in manufacture of dyestuffs and explosives.
- Trinitrotoluene (TNT), use in explosives.
- Mercaptans, used in manufacture of pesticides and as odorizers for hazardous odorless gases.
- 2-nitropropane, used as a solvent.

Spleen. The spleen filters bacteria and particulate matter (especially deteriorated red blood cells) from the blood. Iron is recovered from the hemoglobin for recycling. In the embryo, the spleen forms all types of blood cells. In the adult, however, it produces only certain kinds of leukocytes. Examples of chemicals that damage the spleen are:

- Chloroprene, used in production of synthetic rubber.
- Nitrobenzene, used as chemical intermediate.

Reproductive System. Experimental results indicate that certain agents interfere with the reproductive capabilities of both sexes, causing sterility, infertility, abnormal sperm, low sperm count, and/or affect hormone activity in animals. Many of these also affect human repoduction. Further study is required to identify reproductive toxins and their effects. Some examples of chemicals that have been implicated in reproductive system toxicity include:

- **Male**: Anesthetic gases (halothane, methoxyflurane) cadmium, mercury, lead, boron, methyl mercury, vinyl chloride)DDT, kepone, chlordane, PCB's dioxin, 2,4-D, 2,4,5-T, caarbaryl, paraquat, dibromochloropropane, ethylene dibromide, benzene, toluene, xylene, ethanol, radiation, heat.

- **Female**: DDT, parathion, carbaryl, diethylstilbestrol (DES), PCB's cadmium methyl mercury, hexafluoroacetime

Types of Toxic Effects

Teratogenic. Teratology is derived from Latin and means the study of monsters. In a modern context, teratology is the study of congenital malformations. Teratology is a relatively new discipline that started in 1941 with the correlation of German measles to birth defects. In the 1960s, the first industrial link to teratogens was discovered. The chemical involved was methyl mercury.

The following conditions have associated with **congenital malformations**: Heredity, maternal diseases such as German measles and viral infections during pregnancy, maternal malnutrition, physical injury, radiation, and exposure to chemicals.

Most major structural abnormalities occur during the embryonic period, 5-7 weeks, while physiologic and minor defects occur during the fetal period, 8-36 weeks. Studies using lab animals show the need to evaluate exposure of chemicals for each day of pregnancy. Thalidomide, for example, caused birth defects in rats only when administered during the 12th day of gestation.

A number of chemicals are reactive or can be activated in the body during the gestation period. The degree and nature of the fetal effects then depend upon:

- Developmental state of embryo or fetus when chemical is administered.
- Dose of chemical, route, and exposure interval.
- Transplacental absorption of chemical and levels in tissues of embryo/fetus.
- Ability of maternal liver and placenta to metabolize or detoxify chemical.
- Biologic half-life of chemical or metabolites.
- State of cell cycle when chemical is at toxic concentrations.
- Capacity of embryonic/fetal tissues to detoxify or bioactivate chemicals.
- Ability of damaged cells to repair or recover.

Teratogenic potential has been suggested by animal studies under various conditions:

- Dietary deficiency: Vitamins A, D, E, C, riboflavin, thiamine, nicotinamide, frolic acid, zinc, manganese, magnesium cobalt.

- Hormonal deficiency: Pituitary, thyroxin, insulin.
- Hormonal excess: Cortisone, thyroxin, insulin androgens, estrogens, epinephrine.
- Hormone and vitamin antagonists: 3-acetylpyridine, 6-aminonicotinamide, thiouracils.
- Vitamin excess: Vitamin A, nicotinic acid.
- Antibiotics: Penicillin, tetracyclines, streptomycin.
- Heavy metals: Methyl mercury, mercury salts, lead, thallium, selenium, chelating agents.
- Azo dyes: Trypan blue, Evans blue, Niagara sky blue 6%.
- Producers of anoxia: Carbon monoxide, carbon dioxide.
- Chemicals: Quinine, thiadiazole, salicylate, 2,3,7,8-TCDD, caffeine, nitrosamines, hydroxyurea, boric acid, insecticides, pesticides, DMSO chloroform, carbon tetrachloride, benzene, xylene, cyclohexanone propylene glycol, acetamides, formamides, sulfonamides.
- Physical conditions: hypothermia, hyperthermia, radiation, anoxia.
- Infections: Ten viruses (including German measles and cytomegalovirus), syphilis, gonorrhea.

Far fewer agents have been conclusively shown to be teratogenic in humans: anesthetic gases, organic mercury compounds, ionizing radiation, german measles, and thalidomide.

Mutagenic. Mutagens are agents that cause changes (mutations) in the genetic code, altering DNA. The changes can be chromosomal breaks, rearrangement of chromosome pieces, gain or loss of entire chromosomes, or a change within a gene.

Among agents shown to be mutagenic in humans are:

- Ethylene oxide, used in hospitals as a sterilant.
- Ethyleneimine, an alkylating agent.
- Ionizing radiation.
- Hydrogen peroxide, a bleaching agent.
- Benzene, a chemical intermediate.
- Hydrazine, used in rocket fuel.

The concern over mutagenic agents covers more than the effect that could be passed into the human gene pool (germinal or reproductive cell mutations).

There is also interest in the possibility that some cell mutations may produce carcinogenic of teratogenic responses.

Carcinogenic.   Two types of carcinogenic mechanisms have been identified.

- **Genotoxic**:   Electrophilic carcinogens that alter genes through interaction with DNA. There are three types:

  - Direct or primary carcinogens: Chemicals that act without any bioactivation – for example, bis (chloromethyl) ether, ethylene dibromide, and dimethyl sulfate.
  - Procarcinogens: Chemicals that require biotransformation to activate them to a carcinogen – for example, vinyl chloride and 2-naphthylamine.
  - Inorganic carcinogen: Some of these are preliminarily categorized as genotoxic due to potential for DNA damage. Other compounds in the group may operate through epigenetic mechanisms.

- **Epigenetic**: These are carcinogens that do not act directly with genetic material. Several types are possible:

  - Cocarcinogen: Increases the overall response of a carcinogen when they are administered together – for example, sulfur dioxide, ethanol, and catechol.
  - Promoter: Increases response of a carcinogen when applied after the carcinogen but will not induce cancer by itself – for example, phenol, dithranol.
  - Solid-state: Works by unknown mechanism, but physical form vital to effect (asbestos, metal foils).
  - Hormone: Usually is not genotoxic, but alters endocrine balance; often acts as propoter (DES, estrogens).
  - Immunosuppressor: Mainly stimulates virally induced, transplanted, or metastatic neoplasms by weakening host's immune system (antilymphocytic serum, used in organ transplants).

Genotoxiic carcinogens are sometimes effective after a single exposure can act in a cumulative manner, or act with other genotoxic carcinogens which affect the same organs. Some epigenetic carcinogens, however, only cause cancers when concentrations are high and exposure long. The implication is that while there may be a "safe" threshold level of exposure for some carcinogens, others may have "zero" threshold – that is, one molecule of the chemical can induce a cancer.

Various considerations indicate that **DNA** is a critical target for carcinogens:

- Many carcinogens are or can be metabolized so that they react with DNA. In these cases, the reaction can usually be detected by testing for evidence of DNA repair.
- Many carcinogens are also mutagens.
- Inhibitors and inducers of carcinogens affect mutagenic activity.
- Chemicals often are tested for mutagenic and carcinogenic activity in the same cell systems.
- Defects in DNA repair predispose to cancer development.
- Several inheritable or chromosomal abnormalities predispose to cancer development.
- Initiated dormant tumor cells persist, which is consistent with a change in DNA.
- Cancer is inheritable at the cellular level and, therefore, may result from an alteration of DNA.
- Most, if not all, cancers display chromosomal abnormalities.

Although cancer ranks as the second most common cause of death in the United States, the process of carcinogenesis is not yet clearly defined. As a result, there are several problems encountered when evaluating the carcinogenic potential of various agents in the environment. First, human health can be affected by a wide range of factors, including the environment, occupation, genetic predisposition and lifestyle (i.e., cigarette smoking, diet). Therefore, it is often difficult to determine the relationship between any one exposure and the onset of cancer. Second, many cancers are latent responses – that is, the disease may not be manifested until many years after the initial exposure. Third, the mechanisms for carcinogenesis may differ according to the type and the site of the cancer.

EXPOSURE GUIDELINES

It is necessary, during response activities involving hazardous materials, to acknowledge and plan for the possibility that response personnel will be exposed to the materials present at some time and to some degree. Most materials have levels of exposure that can be tolerated wtihout adverse health effects. However, it is most important to identify the materials involved and then determine: (1) the exposure levels considered safe for each of these materials; (2) the type and extent of exposure; and (3) possible health effects of overexposure.

Several reference sources are available that contain information about toxicological properties and safe exposure limits for many different materials. These sources can be grouped into two general categories: 1) sources that provide toxicological data and general health hazard information and warnings and 2) sources that describe specific legal exposure limits or recommended exposure guidelines.

Both types of sources, considered together, provide useful information that can be used to assess the exposure hazards that might be present at a hazardous materials incident. In the following discussion, these sources are described in greater detail.

General Guidelines

The effects of chemical exposure with the route and dosage required can be found in NIOSH's <u>Registry of Toxic Effects of Chemical Substances</u>. However, because most of the data is for animal exposures, there may be problems in trying to use the data for human exposure guidelines.

Other sources give some general guides on chemical exposure. They may say that the chemical is an irritant or corrosive, or they may give a warning like "AVOID CONTACT" or "AVOID BREATHING VAPORS." This gives the user information about the possible route of exposure and effects of the exposure. However, this does not give a safe exposure limit. One may question if the warning means to "AVOID <u>ANY POSSIBLE</u> CONTACT" or if there is a certain amount that a person can contact safely for a certain length of time.

Two sources of information go a little further and use a ranking system for exposure to chemicals. Irbing Sax, in <u>Dangerous Properties of Industrial Materials</u>, gives a Toxic Hazard Rating (THR) for certain chemicals. These ratings are NONE, LOW, MODERATE, and HIGH. The route of exposure is also given. For example, butylamine is listed as a HIGH toxic hazard via oral and dermal routes and a MODERATE toxic hazard via inhalation. HIGH means that the chemical is "capable of causing death or permanent injury due to the exposures of normal use; incapacitating and poisonous; requires special handling."

In the book, <u>Fire Protection Guide on Hazardous Materials</u>, the National Fire Protection Association (NFPA) also uses a ranking system to identify the toxic hazards of a chemical. These numbers are part of the NFPA 704 M identification system. The numbers used range from 0 to 4 where 0 is for "materials which, on exposure under fire conditions, would offer no health hazard beyond that of ordinary compustible material" and 4 is for materials where "a few whiffs of the gas or vapor could cause death; or the gas, vapor, or liquid could be fatal on penetrating the fire fighters' normal full protective clothing, which is designed for resistance to heat." The degree of hazard is based upon the inherent properties of the chemical and the hazard that could exist under fire or other emergency conditions. This rating is based on an exposure of "a few seconds to an hour" and the possibility of large quantities of material being present. Thus, it is not completely applicable to long-term exposure to small quantities of chemicals. It is more useful for spills or fires where a person could come in contact with a large amount of the chemical.

The Sax and NFPA sources provide information about the routes of exposures and some effects along with a rating system that indicates which chemicals require extra precaution and special protective equipment.

Sources for Specific Guidelines for Airborne Contaminants

While there are many sources for general exposure guidelines, there are only a few that give more specific information about what is considered a safe exposure limit. Many of the following organizations have exposure guidelines for exposures to hazards other than airborne contaminants (e.g., heat stress, noise, radiation). This part will deal only with chemical exposures.

American Conference of Governmental Industrial Hygienists (ACGIH). One of the first groups to develop specific exposure guidelines was the American Conference of Governmental Industrial Hygienists (ACGIH). ACGIH suggested the development of Maximum Allowable Concentrations (MACs) for use by industry. A list of MACs was compiled by ADGIH and published in 1946. In the early 1960s, ACGIH revised those recommendations and renamed them Threshold Limit Values (TLVs®).

Along with the TLVs, ACGIH publishes Biological Exposure Indices (BEIs). BEIs are intended to be used as guides for evaluation of exposure where inhalation is not the only possible route of exposure. Since the TLVs are for inhalation only, they may not be protective if the chemical is ingested or is absorbed through the skin. Biological monitoring (e.g., urine samples, breath analysis) can be used to assess the overall exposure. This monitoring uses information about what occurs in the body (e.g., metabolism of benzene to phenol) to determine if there has been an unsafe exposure. The BEIs serve as a reference for biological monitoring just as TLVs serve as a reference for air monitoring.

The TLVs are reviewed yearly and are published in their booklet, <u>Threshold Limit Values and Biological Exposure Indices</u>.

American National Standards Institute (ANSI). The American National Standards Institute (ANSI) has published standards that are a consensus of the people who have a concern about the subject the standard covers (e.g., hardhats, respirators). An ANSI standard is intended as a guide to aid manufacturers, consumers, and the general public. ANSI has standards covering many aspects of the working environment. Many of these have been adopted by OSHA (see later discussion) as legal requirements.

\Some of the standards were exposre guidelines. They gave "acceptable concentrations", which were "concentrations of air contaminants to which a person may be exposed without discomfort or ill effects." These exposure limits were withdrawn in 1982. However, some were adopted by OSHA before the withdrawal and still may be in use.

Occupational Safety and Health Administration (OSHA). In 1971, the Occupational Safety and Health Administration (OSHA) promulgated Permissible Exposure Limites (PELs). These limits were extracted from the 1968 TLVs, the ANSI standards, and other Federal standards. The PELs are found in 29 CFR 1910.1000. Since then, additional PELs have been adopted and a few of the originals have been changed. These have been incorporated into specific standards for chemicals (e.g., 29 CFR 1910.1028 – Benzene). There are also standards for thirteen carcinogens in which there is no allowable inhalation exposure.

In 2001, OSHA published major revisions to the PELs. Since only a few of the PELs had been updated since 1971, it was decided to update the entire list of PELs by changing existing ones and adding new ones. Again, OSHA looked to the TLVs, but also considered recommendations from the National Institute for Occupational Safety and Health (NIOSH).

Since OSHA is a regulatory agency, their PELs are legally enforceable standards and apply to all private industries and federal agencies. They may also apply to state and local employees depending upon the state laws.

National Institute for Occupational Safety and Health (NIOSH). The National Institute for Occupational Safety and Health (NIOSH) was formed at the same time as OSHA to act as a research organization. IT is charged in part, with making recommendations for new standards and revising old ones as more information is accumulated. The exposure levels NIOSH has researched have been used to develop new OSHA standards, but there are many Recommended Exposure Limits (RELs) that have not been adopted. Thus, they are in the same status as the exposure guidelines of ACGIH and other groups. The RELs are found in the "NIOSH Recommendations for Occupational Health standards" (see Appendix II).

American Industrial Hygiene Association (AIHA). The American Industrial Hygiene Association has provided guidance for industrial hygienists for many years In 1994, AIHA developed exposure guidelines that it calls Workplace Environmental Exposure Level Guides (WEELs). These are reviewed and updated each year. Appendix III has the current list of WEELs. While the list is not as large as others, AIHA has cosen chemicals for which other groups do not have exposure guidelines. Thus, they are providing information to fill the gaps left by others.

<u>Types of Exposure Guidelines</u>

Several organizations develop exposure guidelines. However, the types of guidelines they produce are similar.

Time Weighted Average (TWA). This exposure is determined by averaging the concentrations of the exposure with each concentration weighted based on the duration of exposure. For example, an exposure to acetone at the following concentrations and durations:

> *1000 ppm for 3 hours*
> *500 ppm for2 hours*
> *200 ppm for 3 hours*
> *would have an 8-hour time weighted average exposure of:*

$$\frac{(3 \; hrs) \; (1000 \; ppm) + (2 \; hrs)(500 \; ppm) + (3 \; hrs)(200 \; ppm)}{8 \; hrs}$$

$$= \frac{3000 \; ppm + 1000 \; ppm + 600 \; ppm}{8}$$

$$= \quad 575 \; ppm$$

This exposure would be compared to an 8-hour TWA **exposure limit**.

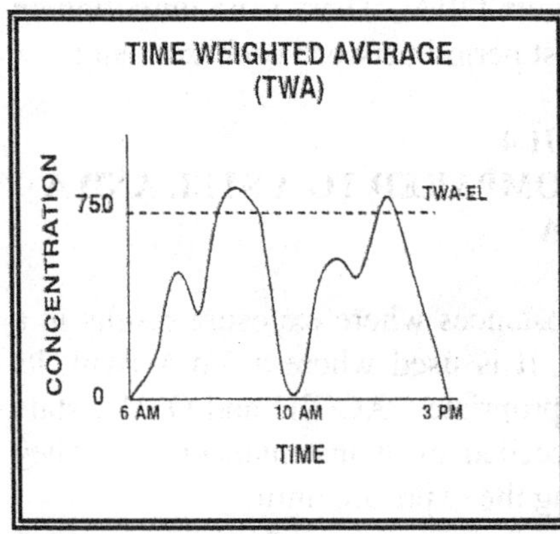

A TWA can be the average concentration over any period of time. However, most TWAs are the average concentration of a chemical most workers can be exposed to during a 40-hour week and a normal 8-hour work day without showing any toxic effects. NIOSH TWA recommendations, on the other hand, can also be based on exposures up to 10 hours. The time weighted average permits exposure to concentrations above the limit, when they are compensated by equal exposure below the TWA. **(GRAPH 3)** shows an example that illustrates this point for a chemical with a TWA exposure limit of 750 ppm.

GRAPH 3
**EXAMPLE OF AN EXPOSURE COMPARED TO A TWA
EXPOSURE LIMIT**

Short Term Exposure Limit (STEL). The excursions allowed by the TWA could involve very high concentrations and cause an adverse effect, but still be within the allowable average. Therefore, some organizations felt that there was a need for a limit to these excursions. In 1976, ACGIH added STELs to its TLVs. The STEL is a 15-minute time-weighted average exposure. Excursions to the STEL should be at least 60 minutes apart, no longer than 15 minutes in duration and should not be repeated more than four times per day. Because the excursions are calculated into the 8-hour

TWA, the exposure must be limited to avoid exceeding the tWA. **GRAPH 4** illustrates an exposure that exceeds the 15-minute limit for a STEL of 1000 ppm.

The STEL supplements the TWA. It reflects an exposure limit that protests against acute effects from a substance that primarily exhibits chronic toxic effects. This concentration is set at a level to protect workers against irritation, narcosis, and irreversible tissue damage. OSHA added STELs to its PELs with the 1989 revisions.

AIHA has some short-term TWAs similar to the STELs. The times used vary from 1 to 30 minutes. These Short-Term TWAs are used in conjunction with, or in place of, the 8-hour TWA. There is no limitation on the number of these excursions or the rest period between each excursion.

GRAPH 4
EXAMPLE OF AN EXPOSURE COMPARED TO A STEL AND A TWA

Ceiling ©. Ceiling values exist for substances where exposure results in a rapid and particular type of response. It is used where a TWA (with its allowable excursions) would not be appropriate. ACGIH and OSHA state that a ceiling value should not be exceeded even instantaneously. They denote a ceiling value by a "C" preceding the exposure limit.

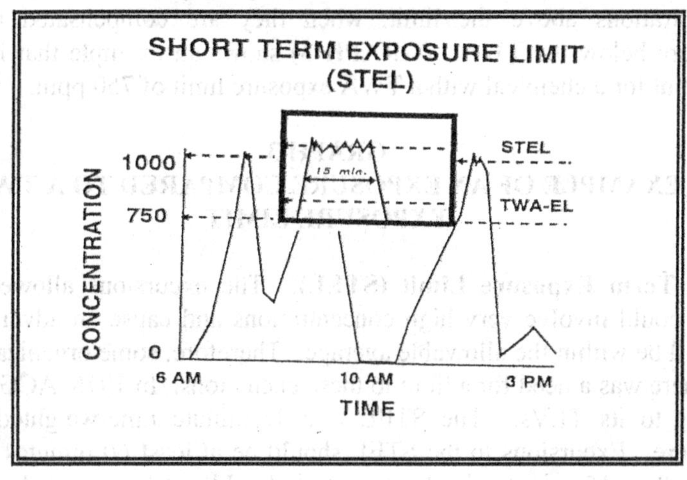

NIOSH also uses ceiling values. However, their ceiling values are more like a STEL. Many have time limits (from 5 to 60 minutes) associated with the exposure. **GRAPH 5** illustrates an exposure that does not exceed a ceiling value of 5 ppm.

GRAPH 5
EXAMPLE OF AN EXPOSURE COMPARED TO A CEILING EXPOSRE LIMIT

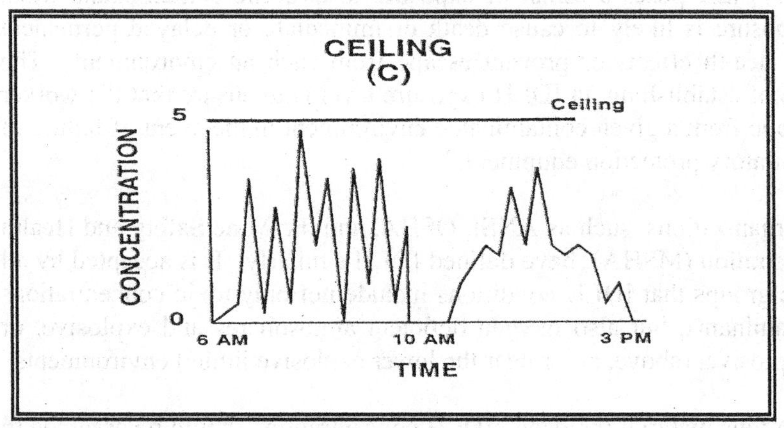

Peaks. Until recently ANSI, and OSHA where they have adopted ANSI standards, had used a peak exposure limit. This peak exposure is an allowable excursion above their ceiling values. The duration and number of exposures at this peak value is limited. For example, ANSI allowed the 25 ppm ceiling value for benzene to be exceeded to 50 ppm but only for 10 minutes during an 8-hour period. ANSI withdrew its exposure limit standards in 1982. With the revision of the PELs in 1989, OSHA has dropped most of its peak values.

"Skin" Notation. While these exposure guidelines are based on exposure to airborne concentrations of chemicals, OSHA, NIOSH, ACGIH, and AIHA recognize, however, that there are other routes of exposure in the workplace. In particular, there can be a contribution to the overall exposure from skin contact with chemicals that can be absorbed through the skin. Unfortunately, there is very little data available that quantifies the amount of allowable skin contact. But some organizations provide qualitative information about skin absorbable chemicals. When a chemical has the potential to contribute to the overall exposure by direct contact with the skin, mucous membranes or eyes, it is given a "skin" notation.

This "skin notation not only points out chemicals that are readily absorbed through the skin, but also notes that if there is skin contact, the exposure guideline for inhalation may not provide adequate protection. The inhalation exposure guidelines are designed for exposures only from inhalation. If additional routes of exposure are added, there can be detrimental effects even if the exposure guideline is not exceeded.

Immediately Dangerous to Life or Health (IDLH). IDLH is defined as a condition "that poses a threat of exposure to airborne contaminants when that exposure is likely to cause death or immediate or delayed permanent adverse health effects or prevent escape from such an environment. The purpose of establishing an IDLH exposure level is to ensure that the worker can escape from a given contaminated environment in the event of failure of the respiratory protection equpment."

Other organizations, such as ANSI, OSHA, and the Mine Safety and Health Administration (MSHA), have defined IDLH similarly. It is accepted by all of these groups that IDLH conditions include not only toxic concentrations of contaminants, but also oxygen deficient atmospheres and explosive, or near-explosive, (above, at, or near the lower explosive limits) environments.

At hazardous material incidents, IDLH concentrations should be assumed to represent concentrations above which only workers wearing respirators that provide the maximum protection (i.e., a positive-pressure, full-facepiece, self-contained breathing apparatus [SCBA] or a combination positive-pressure, full-facepiece, supplied-air respirator with positive-pressure escape (SCBA) are permitted. Specific IDLH concentrations values for many substances can be found in the NIOSH "Pocket Guide to Chemical Hazards." Guidelines for potentially explosive, oxygen deficient, or radioactive environments can be found in the U.S. EPA "Standard Operating Safety Guidelines" and the NIOSH/OSHA/USCG/EPA <u>Occupational Safety and Health Guidance Manual for Hazardous Waste Site Activities</u>.

<u>Exposure Limits for Chemical Mixtures</u>

The exposure limits that have been discussed are based upon exposure to single chemicals. Since many exposures include more than one chemical, values are adjusted to account for the combination. When the effects of the exposure are considered to be additive, a formula can be used to determine whether total exposure exceeds the limits. The calculation used is:

$$E_m = (C_1 \div L_1 + C_2 \div L_2) + \ldots (C_n \div L_n)$$

where: E_m is the equivalent exposure for the mixture.
C is the concentration of a particular contaminant.
L is the exposure limit for that substance.
The value of E_m should not exceed unity (1).

An example using this calculation would be as follows:

Chemical A   C = 200 ppm   L = 750 ppm
Chemical B   C = 100 ppm   L = 500 ppm
Chemical C   C = 50 ppm   L = 200 ppm

$$E_m = 200 \div 750 + 100 \div 500 + 50 \div 200$$
$$E_m = .027 + 0.20 + 0.25$$
$$E_m = 0.72$$

Since E_m is less than unity, the exposure combination is within acceptable limits.

This calculation applies to chemicals where the effects are the same and are additive.   If the combination is not additive, the calculation is not appropriate.

Application of Exposure Guidelines

In 29 CFR 1910.120, "Hazardous Waste Operations and Emergency Response" standard, OSHA specifies the use of certain exposure limits. The exposure limits specified are OSHA's permissible exposure limits (PELs) and "published exposure levels." The "published exposure levels" are used when no PEL exists. A "published exposure level" is defined as "the exposure limits published in 'NIOSH Recommendations for Occupational Health Standards'. If none is specified, the exposure limits published in the standards specified by the American Conference of Governmental Industrial Hygienists in their publication 'Threshold Limit Values and Biological Exposure Indices.'"

Engineered Controls and Work Practices. 29 CVR 1910.120(g)(1)(i) states, "Engineering controls and work practices <u>shall</u> be instituted to reduce and maintain employee exposure to or below the <u>permissible exposure limits</u> for substances regulated by 29 CFR Part 1910, to the extent required by Subpart Z, except to the extent that such controls and practices are not feasible." (emphasis added) Whenever engineering controls and work practices are not feasible, personal protective equipment shall be used to reduce and maintain exposures.

For those substances or hazards where there is no PEL, the published exposure levels, published literature and MSDS will be used for evaluation. In these circumstances, a combination of engineering controls, work practices and PPE shall be used to reduce and maintain exposures.

Personal Protective Equipment. Since PPE must be selected based on the hazards present at the site, the exposure limits are used to evaluate the effectiveness of the PPE. Comparing the actual or expected exposure to the PEL or other exposure limits gives the wearer information on selection of the proper PPE.

Medical Surveillance. 29 CFR 1910.120(f)(2)(i) requires a medical surveillance program for all employees exposed to substances or hazards above the PEL for 30 or more days per year. If there is no PEL, then the published exposure levels are used for evaluation. The exposures are considered even if a respirator was being used at the time of exposure.

<u>Limitations/Restrictions of Exposure Guideline Use</u>

The exposure guidelines discussed in this part are based on industrial experience, experimental human studies, experimental animal studies, or a combination of the three. The guidelines were developed for workers in the industrial environment. Thus, they are not meant to be used for other purposes.

"These limits are intended for use in the practice of industrial hygiene as guidelines or recommendations in the control of potential health hazards and for no other use, e.g., in the evaluation or control of community air pollution nuisances, in estimating the toxic potential of continuous, uninterrupted exposures or other extended work periods, as proof or disproof of an existing disease or physical condition, or adoption by countries those working conditions differ from thsoe in the United States of

America and where substances and processes differ. These limits are not fine lines between safe and dangerous concentration nor are they a relative index of toxicity, and should not be used by anyone untrained in the discipline of industrial hygiene."

As can be seen from this qualifier, these exposure limits are not intended as exposure limits for exposure by the public.

There is the limitation on the use of the exposure guideline as a relative index of toxicity. This is because the exposure limits are based on different effects for different chemicals. For example, the TLV®-TWA for acetone is chosen to prevent irritation to the eyes and respiratory system. The TLV-TWA for acrlonitrile is chosen to reduce the risk to cancer. Exposures to these chemicals at other concentration levels could lead to other effects. Thus, when evaluating the risk of chemical exposure, all toxicological data should be consulted.

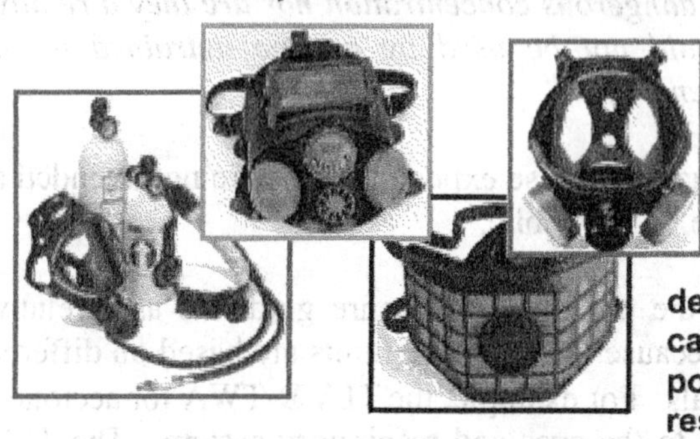

The respiratory system is able to tolerate exposures to toxic gases, vapors, and particulates, but only to a limited degree. Some chemicals can impair or destroy portions of the respiratory tract, or they may be absorbed directly into the bloodstream from the lungs. Chemicals that enter the blood may eventually affect the function of other organs and tissues. The respiratory system can be protected by avoiding or minimizing exposure to harmful substances. Engineering controls such as ventilation help decrease exposure. When these methods are not feasible, respirators may provide protection. Certain respirators can filter gases, vapors, and particulates in the ambient atmosphere, other respirators are available that can supply clean breathing air to the wearer.

The use of respirators is regulated by the Occupational Safety and Health Administration (OSHA) Regulations stipulate the use of approved respirators, proper selection, and individual fitting of respirator users.

Respiratory protection must be used when the concentration of a substance in the ambient atmosphere exceeds a personal exposure limit. Several exposure limits used to determine the need for respiratory protection. In order of precedence, these are the OSHA Permissible Exposure Limits (PELs), NIOSH Recommended Exposure Limits (RELs), and the ACGIH Threshold Limit Values (TLVs). If none of these are available, other published data may be used.

Respiratory Hazards

The normal atmosphere consists of 78% nitrogen, 21% oxygen, 0.9% inert gases and 0.04% carbon dioxide. An atmosphere containing toxic contaminants, even at very low concentrations, could be a hazard to the lungs and body. A concentration large enough to decrease the percentage of oxygen in the air can lead to asphyxiation, even if the contaminant is an inert gas.

Oxygen Deficiency. The body requires oxygen to live. If the oxygen concentration decreases, the body reacts in various ways (TABLE 1). Death occurs rapidly when the concentration decreases to 6%.

Physiological effects of oxygen deficiency are not apparent until the concentration decreases to 16%. The various regulations and standards dealing with respirator use recommend that concentrations ranging from 16-19.5% be considered indicative of an oxygen deficiency. Such numbers take into account individual physiological responses, errors in measurement, and other safety considerations. In hazardous materials response operations, 19.5% oxygen in air is considered the lowest "safe" working concentration. Below 19.5% available oxygen, a supplied air respirator must be used.

TABLE 1 PHYSIOLOGICAL EFFECT OF OXYGEN DEFICIENCY	
% Oxygen (by volume) at Sea Level	Effects
21-16	Nothing abnormal
16-12	Loss of peripheral vision, increased breathing volume, accelerated heartbeat, impaired attention and thinking, impaired coordination.
12-10	Very faulty judgment, very poor muscular coordination, muscular exertion causes fatigue that may cause permanent heart damage, intermittent respiration.
10-6	Nausea, vomiting, inability to perform vigorous movement, or loss of all movement, unconsciousness, followed by death.
< 6	Spasmatic breathing, convulsive movements, death in minutes

Aerosols. Aerosol is a term used to describe fine particulates (solid or liquid) suspended in air. Particulates ranging in diameter from 5 to 30 microns are deposited in the nasal and pharyngeal passages. The trachea and smaller conducting tubes collect particulates 1-5 microns in diameter. For particulates to diffuse from the bronchioles into alveoli, they must be less than 0.5 microns in diameter. Large particles do reach the alveoli due to gravity. The smallest particulates may never be deposited in the alveoli and so may diffuse back into the conducting tubes to be exhaled.

Aerosols can be classified in two ways: by their physical form and origin and by the physiological effect on the body.

- • Physical Classification Examples
     Mechanical dispersoid: liquid or solid particle
          mechanically produced.
  - ✓ Condensation dispersoid: liquid or solid particle
          often produced by combustion.
  - ✓ Spray: visible liquid mechanical dispersoid.
  - ✓ Fume: extremely small solid condensation dispersoid.
  - ✓ Mist: liquid condensation dispersoid.
  - ✓ Fog: mist dense enough to obscure vision.
  - ✓ Smoke: liquid or solid organic particles resulting from
  - ✓ Incomplete combustion.
  - ✓ Smog: mixture of smoke and fog.
- • Physiological Classification Examples:
  - ✓ Nuisance: no lung injury but proper lung
          functioning inhibited.
  - ✓ Inert pulmonary reaction causing: non-specific reaction
  - ✓ Pulmonary fibrosis causing: effects ranging from nodule
  - ✓ production in lungs to serious diseases such as
          asbestosis.
  - ✓ Chemical irritation: irritation, inflammation, or ulceration of lung tissue.
  - ✓ Systemic poison: diseases in other parts of the body.
  - ✓ Allergy-producing: causes allergic hypersensitivity reactions
  - ✓ such as itching or sneezing.

Gaseous Contaminants. Gases and vapors are filtered to some degree on their trip through the respiratory tract. Soluble gases and vapors are absorbed by the conducting tubes en route to the alveoli. Not all will be absorbed so that along with insoluble gases, they finally diffuse into the alveoli where they can be directly absorbed into the bloodstream.

Gaseous contaminants can be classified as chemical and physiological hazards.
- • Chemical Contaminants:

- Acidic: acids or react with water to form acids.
- Alkaline: bases or react with water to
- form bases.
- Organic: compounds that contain carbon; may
- range from methane to chlorinated organic
- solvents.
- Organometallic: organic compounds containing
- metals.
- Hydrides: compound in which hydrogen is
- bonded to another metal.
- Inert: no chemical reactivity.

- **Physiological Contaminants:**
  Irritants: corrosive substances that injury and
  inflame tissue.
  Asphyxiants: substances that displace oxygen or prevent the use of oxygen in the body.
  Anesthetics: substances that depress the central nervous system, causing a loss of sensation or intoxication.
  Systemic poisons: substances that can cause disease in arious organ systems.

Respirator Use and Selection

The health of a respirator wearer is based on how the respirator is used.

The Occupational Safety and Health Administration (OSHA), in 29 CFR Part 1910.120, refers to 29 CFR Part 1910.134 as the source of respiratory protection regulations issued in 2001. In 29 CFR Part 1910.134,

Section b of 29 CFR 1910.134, requires a "minimal acceptable program" to ensure sound respiratory protection practices. The balance of the regulations discusses specific requirements for respiratory use. The requirements for a minimal acceptable program are quoted from 29 CFR 1910.134 as follows:

- Written standard operating procedures governing the selection and use of respirators shall be established.

- Respirators shall be selected on the basis of the hazards to which the worker is exposed.
- The user shall be instructed and trained in the proper use of respirators and their limitations.
- Respirators shall be regularly cleaned and disinfected. Those used by more than one worker shall be thoroughly cleaned and disinfected after each use.
- Respirators shall be stored in a convenient, clean, and sanitary location.
- Respirators used routinely shall be inspected during cleaning. Worn or deteriorated parts shall be replaced. Respirators for emergency use such as self-contained devices shall be thoroughly inspected at least once a month and after each use.
- Appropriate surveillance of work area conditions and degree of employee exposure or stress shall be maintained.
- There shall be regular inspection and evaluation to determine the continued effectiveness of the program.
- Persons should not be assigned to tasks requiring the use of respirators unless it has been determined that they are physically able to perform the work and use the equipment. The local physician shall determine what health and physical conditions are pertinent. The respirator user's medical status should be reviewed periodically (for instance annually).
- Approved respirators shall be used. The respirator furnished shall provide adequate respiratory protection against the particular hazard for which it is designed in accordance with approvals established by the National Institute for Occupational Safety and Health (NIOSH).

In general OSHA states that the selection of the proper approved respirator depends upon:

- The nature of the hazard.
- The characteristics of the hazardous operation or process.
- The location of the hazardous area with respect to a safe area having respirable air.
- The period of time for which respiratory protection may be needed.
- The activity of workers in the hazardous area.
- The physical characteristics, functional capabilities and limitations of respirators of various types.
- The respirator/protection factors and respirator fit.

All of these criteria must be considered in the selection of a respirator.

<u>Respirator Approval</u>

OSHA regulations require the use of approved respirators. Respirators are tested by NIOSH in accordance with the requirements of 30 CFR Part 11.

An NIOSH approval indicates that the respirator in use is identical to the one submitted for the original approval. If a manufacturer changes any part of the respirator without resubmitting it to the NIOSH Testing Lab, the approval is invalid and will be rescinded. This is intended to protect the respirator user. Also, any unauthorized changes or hybridization of a respirator by the user invalidates the respirator approval and all the guarantees understood with the approval.

NIOSH is responsible for respirator certification. Thus respirators in use today must bear approval numbers by NIOSH. The approval number must be displayed on the respirator or its container. It consists of the prefix TC (Testing and Certification), the schedule number, followed by the approval number. For example in TC-13F-69, "13" is the schedule for self-contained breathing apparatus, "F" indicates the number of revisions to the schedule, and 69 is the consecutive approval number. Also, the approval label includes the certifying agencies.

Periodically, NIOSH publishes a list of all approved respirators and respirator components. NIOSH Publication No. 91-101 document is used to answer two basic questions about respiratory protection:

- Is this respirator appropriate (approved) for the existing work conditions?
- Is this respirator (mask and purifying elements) an approved assembly?

If the answer to either of these questions is "no," then the worker is prohibited from using that respirator (or type of respirator).

AIR-PURIFYING RESPIRATORS

Air-Purifying Respirators (APRs) refer to respirators that remove contaminants by passing the breathing air through a purifying element. There is a wide variety of APRs available to protect against specific contaminants but they all fall into two subclasses: (1) particulate APRs that employ a mechanical filter element, and (2) gas and vapor removing APRs that utilize chemical sorbents contained in a cartridge or canister.

Air-purifying respirators may be used only if all of the following requirements are met:

- The identity and concentration of the contaminant are known.
- The ambient concentration of a contaminant is below the Immediately Dangerous to Life or Health (IDLH) concentration.
- The oxygen content in the atmosphere is greater than 19.5%
- The respirator assembly is approved for protection against the specific concentration of a contaminant.
- There is periodic monitoring of the work area.
- The respirator assembly has been successfully fit-tested on the user.

Requirements for APR Use

The use of an air-purifying respirator is contingent upon a number of criteria. If the conditions spelled out in this section of the text cannot be met, then use of an APR is prohibited.

- Oxygen Content. The normal atmosphere contains approximately 21% oxygen. The physiological effects of reduced oxygen begin to be evident at 16%. Without regard to contaminants, the atmosphere must contain a minimum of 19.5% oxygen to permit use of an air-purifying respirator. This is a legal requirement of 30 CFR Part 11 and a recommendation of ANSI 288.2. Below 19.5% oxygen, atmosphere-supplying respirators must be used instead.

- Identification of Contaminants. It is absolutely imperative that the contaminant(s) be known so that the toxic effects of inhaling the contaminant can be determined; appropriate particulate filters or cartridges/canisters can be chosen; it can be determined that adequate warning properties exist for the contaminant; and, the appropriate facepiece be selected (full-face mask is necessary if the agent causes eye irritation).

- **Known Contaminant Concentration.** The maximum concentration depends on the contaminant and the respirator: the concentration must not exceed IDLH; the Maximum Use Limit of the respirator cannot be exceeded (MUL=APF x EL); the Maximum Use Concentration of a particular type and size cartridge or canister must not be surpassed; and the expected service life (cartridge/canister efficiency) should be determined.

- **Periodic Monitoring of Hazards.** Because of the importance of knowing the identity and concentration of the contaminant(s), monitoring of the work area with appropriate equipment must occur at least periodically during the workday. This is done to ensure that no significant changes have occurred and the respirators being used are adequate for the work conditions.

- **Approval of Respirators.** The respirator assembly (facepiece and air-purifying elements) is approved for protection against the contaminant

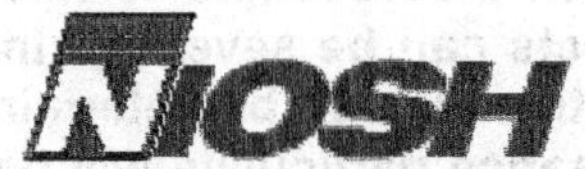

at the concentration which is present in the work area. The concentration must not exceed the NIOSH designated MUC for that type and size cartridge or canister.

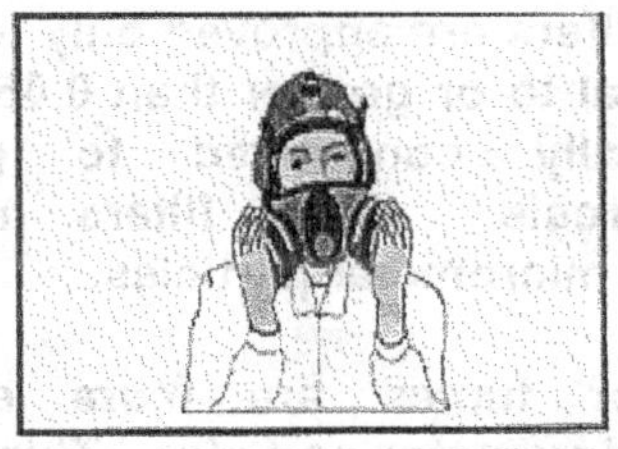

- **Fit-test.** The wearer must pass a qualitative fit-test for the make, model, and size of air-purifying device used. The OSHA regulations, in 29 CFR 910.134(e)(5)(i), state: "Every respirator wearer shall receive fitting instructions including demonstrations and practice in how the respirator is worn, how to adjust it, and how to determine if it fits properly.

Respirators shall not be worn when conditions prevent a good face seal. Such conditions may be growth of beard, sideburns, a skull cap that projects under the facepiece, or temple pieces on glasses. Also, the absence of one or both dentures can seriously affect the fit of a facepiece. The worker's diligence in observing these factors shall be evaluated by periodic check. To assure proper protection, the facepiece fit shall be checked by the wearer each time he puts on the respirator. This may be done by giving fitting instructions."

Air-Purifying Elements

Respiratory hazards can be broken down into two classes: particulates and vapors/gases. Particulates are filtered by mechanical means, while vapors and gases are removed by sorbents that react chemically with them. Respirators using a combination of mechanical filter and chemical sorbent will effectively remove both hazards.

- **Particulate-Removing Filters**

  Particulates can occur as dusts, fumes, or mists. The particle size can range from macroscopic to microscopic, and their toxicological effects can be severe or innocuous. The hazard posed by a particulate can be determined by its exposure limit (EL). A nuisance particulate will have an EL of 10 mg/m^3, while a toxic particulate may have an EL well below 0.05 mg/m^3.

  Mechanical filters are classified according to the protection for which they are approved under schedule 21C of 30 CFR Part 11. Most particulate filters are approved only for dusts and/or mists with ELs equal to or greater than 0.05 mg/m^3. These dusts are usually considered to produce pneumoconiosis and fibrosis. Such filters have an efficiency of 80-90% for 0I6 micrometer particles.

  Respirators approved for fumes are more efficient, removing 90-99% for 0.6 micrometer particles. This type of respirator is approved for dusts, fumes, and mists with ELs equal to or greater than 0.05 mg/m^3.

  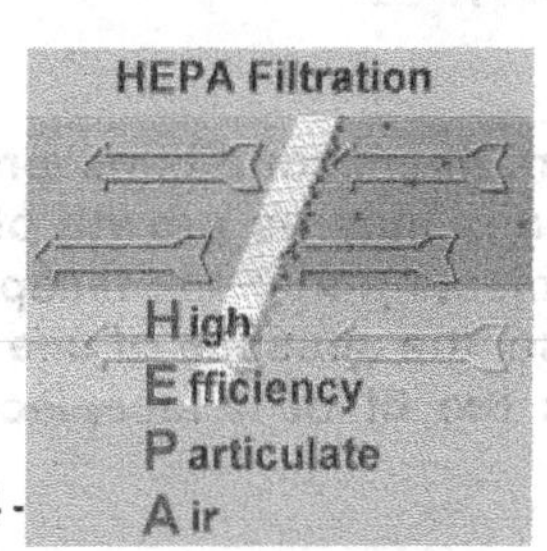

  Finally, there is a high efficiency filter, which is 99.97% effective against particles 0.3 microns in diameter. It is approved for dusts, mists, and fumes with an EL less than 0.05 mg/m^3.

Mechanical filters load with particulates as they are used. As they do, they become more efficient, but also become more difficult to breathe through. When a mechanical filter becomes difficult to breathe through, it should be replaced.

- **Gas and Vapor-Removing Cartridges and Canisters**
  When selecting a gas- or vapor-removing element, it must be chosen for protection against a specific type of contaminant. Some of the commonly employed types of chemical cartridges and canisters and their OSHA-required color coding are listed in the OSHA respirator regulations for general industry (29 CFR 1910.134).

  Gas- and vapor-elements are available in different styles. The physical differences are: (1) size and (2) means of attachment to the facepiece. The smallest elements are cartridges that contain 50-200 cm^3 of sorbent and attach directly to the facepiece, usually in pairs. Chin canisters have a volume of 250-500 cm^3 and are attached to a full facepiece. Gas mask, or industrial-size canisters contain 1000-2000 cm^3 and are attached by a harness to the wearer's front or back and connected to the full-facepiece by a breathing hose.

  The difference in applications is the Maximum Use Concentration (MUC) for which the cartridge or canister can be used in accordance with its NIOSH approval. For example, organic vapors can be removed by the appropriate cartridges, chin canister, or gas-mask canister. Cartridges are approved for use in atmospheres up to 1,000 ppm (0.1%) organic vapors, chin style canisters up to 5000 ppm (0.5%), and gas mask canisters up to 20,000 ppm (2.0%). However, no air-purifying respirator is permitted in an IDLH atmosphere.

  Each sorbent has a finite capacity for removing contaminants and when this limit is reached the cartridge or canister is said to be saturated. At this point, the element will allow the contaminant to pass through and enter the facepiece. The length of time a cartridge or canister will effectively sorb the contaminant is known as the service life of the element. Service life of a type of cartridge or canister is dependent on several factors: the breathing rate of the wearer; contaminant concentration; and sorption efficiency.

TABLE 2 CHEMICAL CARTRIDGE TYPES AND COLOR CODING §1910.134 29 CFR Ch. XVII	
Atmospheric contaminants to be Protected against	**Colors assigned[1]**
Acid gases	White
Hydrocyanic acid gas	White with ½-inch green stripe completely around the canister near the bottom
Chlorine gas	White with ½-inch yellow stripe completely around the canister near the bottom
Organic vapors	Black
Ammonia gas	Green
Acid gases and ammonia gas	Green with ½-inch yellow stripe completely around the canister near the bottom
Carbon monoxide	Blue
Acid gases and organic vapors	Yellow
Hydrocyanic acid gas and chloropicrin vapor	Yellow with ½-inch yellow stripe completely around the canister near the bottom
Acid gases, organic vapors, and ammonia gases	Brown
Radioactive materials, excepting tritium and noble gases	Purple (Magenta)
Particulates (dusts, fumes, mists, fogs, or smokes) in combination with any of the above gases or vapors	Canister color for contaminant, as designated above, with ½-inch gray stripe completely around the canister near the top
All of the above atmospheric contaminants	Red with ½-inch gray stripe completely around the canister near the top

[1] Gray shall not be assigned as the main color for a canister designed to remove acids or vapors.

NOTE: Orange shall be used as a complete body, or stripe color to represent gases not included in this table. The user will need to refer to the canister label to determine the degree of protection the canister will afford.

If the breathing rate of the user is rapid, the flow rate of the contaminated air drawn through the cartridge is greater than it is at a moderate or slow respiration rate. A higher flow rate brings a larger amount of contaminant in contact with the sorbent in a given period of time which, in turn, increases the rate of sorbent saturation and shortens service life.

The expected service life of an organic vapor cartridge decreases as ambient contaminant concentration increases. As concentration goes up, the mass flow rate increases, bringing more contaminant in contact with the sorbent in a given period of time. For example, at any constant breathing rate, ten times as much contaminant contacts the element when the concentration is 500 ppm compared to 50 ppm.

Chemical sorbents vary in their ability to remove contaminants from air. TABLE 3 compares the efficiency of organic vapor cartridges for a number of solvents by recording the amount of time until a 1% breakthrough concentration was measured in the cartridge-filtered air. The initial test concentration is 1000 ppm of solvent vapor; the breakthrough concentration is 10 ppm. From the table, it can be seen that it takes 107 minutes for chlorobenzene to reach a 1% breakthrough, while it only takes 3.0 minutes for vinyl chloride. The sorbent (activated carbon) in the organic vapor cartridge is much better for removing chlorobenzene than vinyl chloride under the test conditions. Cartridge efficiencies need to be considered when selecting and using APRs.

A warning property is used as a sign that a cartridge or canister in use is beginning to lose its effectiveness. A warning property can be detected as an odor, taste, or irritation. At the first such signal, the old cartridge or canister must be exchanged for a fresh one. Without a warning property, respirator efficiency may drop without the knowledge of the wearer, ultimately causing a health hazard.

Most substances have warning properties at some concentration. A warning property detected only at dangerous levels − that is, greater than EL − is not considered adequate. An odor, taste, or irritation detected at extremely low concentrations is also not adequate because the warning is being given all the time or long before the filter begins to lose its effectiveness. In this case, the wearer would never realize when the filter actually becomes ineffective.

The best concentration for a warning property to be first detected is around the EL. For example, toluene has an odor threshold of 40 ppm and an EL of 100 ppm. This is usually considered an adequate warning property. Conversely, dimethylformamide has an EL of 10 ppm and an threshold of 100 ppm. An odor threshold ten times the EL is not an adequate warning property.

If a substance causes rapid olfactory fatigue (that is, the sense of smell is no longer effective), its odor is not an adequate warning property. For example, upon entering an atmosphere containing hydrogen sulfide, the odor is quite noticeable. After a short period of time, it is no longer detectable.

TABLE 3	
EFFECTS OF SOLVENT VAPOR ON RESPIRATOR CARTRIDGE EFFICIENCY	
Solvent	Time to Reach 1% Breakthrough (10 ppm) Minutes
Aromatics	
Benzene	73
Toluene	94
Ethyl benzene	84
m-Xylene	99
Cumene	81
Mestiylene	86
Alcohols	
Menthanol	0.2
Ethanol	28
Isopropanol	54
Allyl alcohol	66
n-Propanol	70
sec-Butanol	96
Butanol	115
2-Methoxyethanol	116
Isoamyl alcohol	97
4-Methyl-2-pentanol	75
2-Ethoxyethanol	77
Amyl alcohol	102
2-Ethyl-1-butanol	76,5
Monochlorides	
Methyl chloride	
Vinyl chloride	0.05
Ethyl chloride	3.8
Allyl chloride	5.6
1-Chloropropane	31
0-Chlorobutane	25
Chlorocyclopentane	72
Chlorobenzene	78
1-Chlorohexane	107
0-Chlorotoluene	77
1-Chloroheptane	102
3-(Chloromethyl heptane)	82
	63

Determining Respirator Protection

The protection provided the wearer is a function of how well the facepiece (mask) fits. No matter how efficient the purifying element, there is little protection afforded if the respirator mask does not provide a leak-free facepiece-to-face seal. Facepieces are available in three basic configurations that relate to their protective capacity:

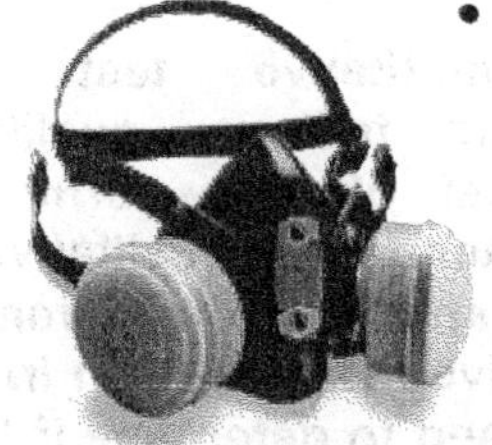

- A quarter-mask fits over the bridge of the nose, along the cheek, and across the top of the chin. The headbands that hold the respirator in place are attached at two or four places of the mask. Limited protection is expected because the respirator can be easily dislocated, creating a breach in the seal.

- A half-mask fits over the bridge of the nose, along the cheek, and under the chin. Headbands have a four-point suspension. Because they maintain a better seal and are less likely to be dislocated, half-masks give better protection than quarter masks.

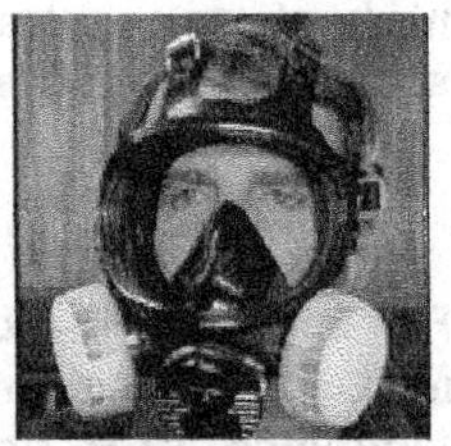

- A full-facepiece fits across the forehead, down over the temples and cheeks, and under the chin. They typically have a head harness with a five or six-point suspension. These masks give the greatest protection because they are held in place more securely and because it is easier to maintain a good seal along the forehead than it is across the top of the nose. An added benefit is the eye protection from the clear lens in the full-facepiece.

The use of respirators is prohibited when conditions prevent a good facepiece-to-face seal. Some examples of these conditions are facial hair, skullcaps, long hair, makeup, temple pieces on eyeglasses. Because maintaining a leak-free seal is so important, personnel required to wear respirators must successfully pass a fit-test designed to check the integrity of the seal. There are two types of fit-tests: quantitative and qualitative. The quantitative test is an analytical determination of the concentration of a test agent inside the facepiece compared to that outside the mask. This concentration ratio is called the Assigned Protection Factor (APF) and is a measure of the relative protection offered by a respirator. For example, if the ambient concentration of the test agent is 1000 and the concentration inside the mask is 10 ppm, the respirator gives the tested individual an APF of 100. So:

$$APF = \frac{\text{Concentration outside mask}}{\text{Concentration inside mask}}$$

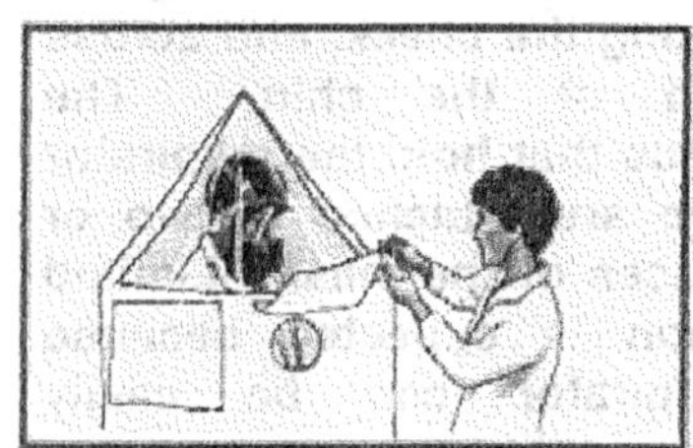

Because quantitative tests are expensive and tedious, qualitative tests are most often performed to check respirator fit. A qualitative fit-test is not an analytical measurement. It is a subjective test where an irritant or aroma is used to determine if there is a good facepiece-to-face seal. If the test subject does not respond (by smelling, tasting, coughing, etc.) to the test agent, he/she can wear the tested respirator with the APF for that type of mask. TABLE 4 lists several types of respirators and their APFs.

A Protection Factor is used to determine the Maximum Use Limit (MUL) of a successfully fit-tested respirator. The MUL is the highest concentration, not exceeding IDLH concentration, of a specific contaminant in which a respirator can be worn:

$$MUL = APF \times TLV$$

For example, if a contaminant has a TLV-TWA of 10 ppm, then the MUL for any half-mask respirator is 100 ppm. The MUL for a full-facepiece APR or demand SCBA is 1000 ppm. If the ambient concentration is greater than 1000 ppm, then a pressure demand SCBA is required because the Maximum Use Concentration (MUC) for organic vapor cartridges is 1000 ppm.

Fit testing and Assigned Protection Factors are only two of the several considerations for selecting the proper type of respirator.

TABLE 4
RESPIRATOR ASSIGNED PROTECTION FACTORS*

Type of Respirator	NIOSH APF (Qualitative Test)
Air-purifying	
quarter-mask	5
half-mask	10
Air-line	
quarter-mask	10
half-mask	10

Hose mask	
full facepiece	10
SCBA, demand	10
quarter-mask	10
half-mask	
Air-purifying	50
full facepiece	
Air-line, demand	50
full facepiece	
SCBA, demand	50
full facepiece	
Air-line, pressure-demand,	
with escape provision	10,000
full facepiece (no test	
required)	
SCBA, pressure-demand or positive pressure	
full facepiece (no test required)	10,000

ATMOSPHERE-SUPPLYING RESPIRATORS

Atmosphere-supplying respirators refer to another classification of respirators. These types of respirators provide a substitute source of breathing air. The respirable air may be supplied to the wearer by a portable breathing air source (a Self-Contained Breathing Apparatus) or by a stationary source such as an air line (a Supplied-Air Respirator).

Types of Atmosphere-Supplying Respirators

Respiratory apparatus must frequently be used during response to hazardous materials incidents. If the contaminant is unknown, or the requirements for using air-purifying respirators cannot be met, then an atmosphere-supplying respirator is required. Several types of atmosphere-supplying devices are available.

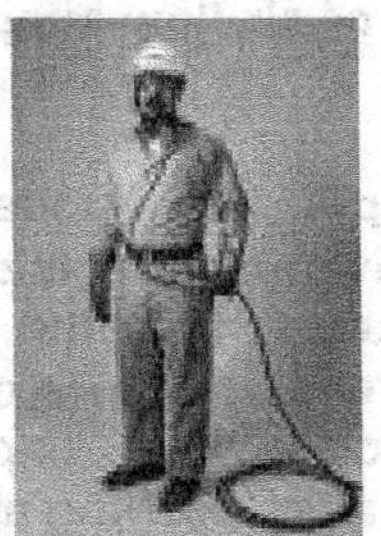

- **Hose Mask.** This type of respirator consists of a facepiece attached to a large diameter hose that transports clean air from a remote area. In units where the wearer breathes the air in, the hose lines can go up to 75 feet. With powered units, the hose length can vary from 50 to 250 feet.

- **Airline Respirator.** The airline respirator is similar to the hose mask, except that breathing-grade air is delivered to the wearer under pressure, either from a compressor or a bank of compressed air cylinders. The air may flow continuously, or it may be delivered as the wearer breathes (demands it). The air source must not be depletable, and no more than 300 feet of airline is allowed. An SCBA escape device is required for entry into an IDLH atmosphere.

- **Oxygen-Generating.** One of the oldest respirators is the oxygen-generating respirator, which utilizes a canister of potassium superoxide. The chemical reacts with water vapor to produce oxygen, which replenishes the wearer's exhaled breath. Exhaled CO_2 is removed by a scrubber device containing LiOH. This reoxygenated air is then returned to the wearer. Oxygen-generating respirators have been used by the military and for escape purposes in mines. It generally is not used for hazardous material applications because of the chemical reaction taking place within the respirator itself.

- **Self-Contained Breathing Apparatus.** The self-contained
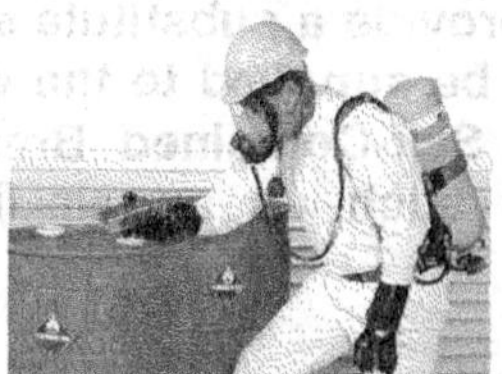
breathing apparatus (SCBA) consists of a facepiece and regulator mechanism connected to a cylinder of compressed air or oxygen carried by the wearer. The SCBA is generally used because it allows the wearer to work without being confined by a hose or air line. The wearer of the SCBA depends on it to supply clean breathing air.

<u>Modes of Operation</u>

The Self-Contained Breathing apparatus and the Supplied-Air Respirator may be differentiated by the type of air flow supplied to the facepiece:

- **Negative-pressure.** In a negative-pressure mode (also referred to as demand mode), a negative pressure is created inside the facepiece and breathing tubes when the wearer inhales (TABLE 5). This negative pressure draws down a diaphragm in the SCBA's regulator. The diaphragm depresses and opens the admission valve, allowing air to be inhaled. As long as the negative pressure remains, air flows to the facepiece.

- **The problem with demand operation is that the wearer can inhale contaminated air through any gaps in the facepiece-to-face sealing surface. Hence, a demand apparatus with a full facepiece is assigned a Protection Factor of only 100, the same as for a full-face air-purifying respirator.

- **Positive-pressure.** In the positive-pressure mode (also referred to as a pressure-demand mode), a positive pressure is maintained inside the facepiece at all times. The system is designed so that the admission valve remains open until enough pressure is built up to close it. The pressure builds up because air is prevented from leaving the system until the wearer exhales. Less pressure is required to close the admission valve than is required to open the spring-loaded exhalation valve.

- At all times, the pressure in the facepiece is greater than the ambient pressure outside the facepiece. If any leakage occurs, it is outward from the facepiece. Because of this, the pressure-demand (positive-pressure) SCBA has been assigned a Protection Factor of 10,000.

TABLE 5		
RELATIVE PRESSURE INSIDE AND OUTSIDE SCBA FACEPIECE		
	Demand	Pressure demand (positive pressure)
Inhalation	-	+
Exhalation	+	+
Static (between breaths)	same	+

Types of SCBAs

There are two types of SCBA apparatus: closed-circuit, which use compressed oxygen, and open-circuit, which use compressed air. SCBAs may operate in one of two modes, demand (negative-pressure) or pressure-demand (positive-pressure). The length of time an SCBA operates is based on the air supply. The units available operate from five minutes to over four hours. The pressure-demand (positive pressure) is the only approved type of open-circuit SCBA for use in hazardous environments by the U.S. EPA and NFPA.

Closed-Circuit SCBA

The closed-circuit SCBA (FIGURE 1, commonly called the rebreather, was developed especially for oxygen-deficient situations. Because it recycles exhaled breath and carries only a small oxygen supply, the service time can be considerably greater than an open-circuit device, which must carry all of the user's breathing air).

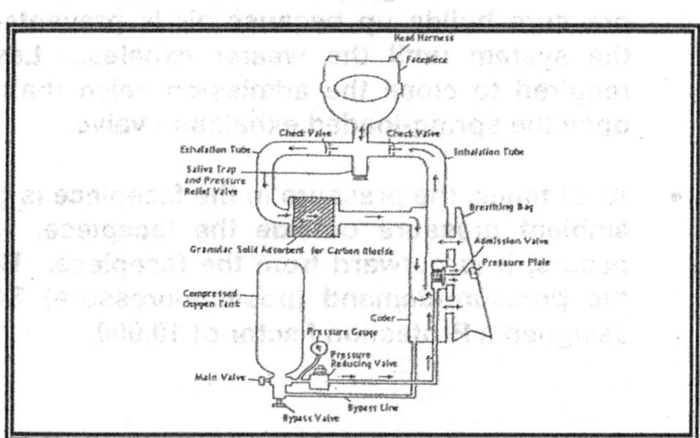

**FIGURE 1
CLOSED-
CIRCUIT
SCBA**

The air for breathing is mixed in a flexible breathing bag. This air is inhaled, deflating the breathing bag. The deflation depresses the admission valve, allowing the oxygen to enter the bag. There it mixes with exhaled breath, from which carbon dioxide has just been removed by passage through a CO_2 scrubber.

Most rebreathers operate in the demand mode. Several rebreathers are designed to provide a positive pressure in the facepiece. The approval schedule 13F under 30 CFR Park II for closed-circuit SCBA makes no provisions for testing "demand" or "pressure-demand" rebreathers. The approval schedule was set up to certify only rebreathers that happen to operate in the demand mode. Thus, rebreathers designed to operate in the positive pressure mode can be approved strictly as closed-circuit apparatus. Since regulations make no distinction, and selection is based on approval criteria, rebreathers designed to maintain a positive pressure can only be considered as a demand-type apparatus. Rebreathers use either compressed oxygen or liquid oxygen. To assure the quality of the air to be breathed, the oxygen must be at least medical grade

breathing oxygen which meets the requirements set by the
"U.S. Pharmacopeia."

- **Open-Circuit SCBA**

  The open-circuit SCBA requires a supply of compressed
  breathing air. The user simply inhales and exhales. The
  exhaled air is exhausted from the system. Because the air
  is not recycled, the wearer must carry the full air supply,
  which limits a unit to the amount of air that the wearer can
  easily carry. Available SCBA's can last from 5 to 60
  minutes. Units that have 5- to 15-minute air supplies are
  only applicable to escape situations.

  The air used in open-circuit apparatus must meet the
  requirements in the Compressed Gas Association's
  Pamphlet G-7.1, which calls for at least "Grade D." Grade D
  air must contain 19.5 to 23.5% oxygen with the balance
  being predominantly nitrogen. Condensed hydrocarbons
  are limited to 5 mg/m^3, carbon monoxide to 20 parts per
  million (ppm) and carbon dioxide to 1,000 ppm. An
  undesirable odor is also prohibited. Air quality can be
  checked using an oxygen meter, carbon monoxide meter,
  and detector tubes.

Components of an Open-Circuit, Positive-Pressure SCBA

The user should be completely familiar with the SCBA being worn.
Checkout procedures have been developed for inspecting an SCBA
prior to use, allowing the user to recognize potential problems. An
individual who checks out the unit is more comfortable and
confident wearing it. If the wearer is not properly trained to wear
the SCBA or it is not properly cared for, then it may fail to provide
the protection expected.

- **Backpack and harness.** A backpack and harness support
  the cylinder and regulator, allowing the user to move freely.
  Weight should be supported on the hips not the shoulders.

- **Cylinder.** Compressed air is considered a hazardous
  material. For this reason, any cylinder used with a SCBA
  must meet the Department of Transportation's (DOT)
  "General Requirements for Shipments and Packaging" (49

CFR Part 173) and "Shipping Container Specification" (49 CFR Part 178).

A hydrostatic test must be performed on a cylinder at regular intervals: for steel and aluminum cylinders, every five years; for composite cylinders (glass fiber/aluminum), every three years. Composite cylinders are relatively new, designed with fiberglass. Composite cylinders have a DOT exemption because there are no set construction requirements at this time. Overall difference is in weight. The construction technology reduces the weight of the cylinder and thereby the overall weight of the SCBA.

Air volume of 45 cubic feet of Grade D air at a pressure of 2,216 pounds per square inch (psi) is needed for a 30-minute supply. Cylinders are filled using a compressor or a cascade system of several large cylinders of breathing air. If the cylinder is overfilled, a rupture disc releases the pressure. The rupture disc is located at the cylinder valve, along with a cylinder pressure gauge to be accurate within ±5%. Because the gauge is exposed and subject to abuse, it should be used only for judging if the cylinder is full, and not for monitoring air supply to the wearer.

- High-Pressure Hose. The high-pressure hose connects the cylinder and the regulator. The hose should be connected to the cylinder only by hand, never with a wrench. An O-ring inside the connector assures a good seal.

- Alarm. A low-pressure warning alarm is located near the connection to the cylinder. This alarm sounds to alert the wearer that only 20-25% of the full cylinder air supply is available for retreat, usually five to eight minutes.

- Regulator Assembly. Air travels from the cylinder through the high-pressure hose to the regulator (FIGURE 2). There it can travel one of two paths. If the bypass valve is opened, air travels directly through the breathing hose into the facepiece. If the mainline valve is opened, air passes through the regulator

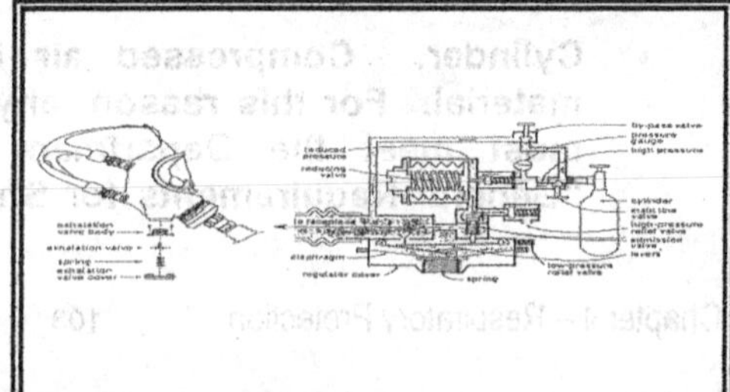

- and is controlled by that mechanism. Also at the regulator (before air enters one of the valves) is another pressure gauge, which also must be accurate to +5%. Because it is visible and well protected, this gauge should be used to monitor the air supply.
- Under normal conditions, the bypass valve is closed and the mainline valve opened so air can center the regulator. Once in the regulator, the air pressure is reduced from the actual cylinder pressure to approximately 50-100 psi by reducing mechanism. A pressure relief valve is located after the pressure reducer for safety should the pressure reducer malfunction.
- Breathing Hose and Facepiece. The breathing hose connects the regulator to the facepiece. Rubber gaskets at both ends provide tight seals. The hose is usually constructed of neoprene and is corrugated to allow stretching.

  Above the point in the mask where the hose is connected, is a one-way check valve. This valve allows air to be drawn from the hose when the wearer inhales but prevents exhaled air from entering the breathing hose. If the check valve is not in place, the exhaled air may not be completely exhausted from the facepieces.

The facepiece is normally constructed of neoprene, but sometimes of silicone rubber. Five- or six-point suspension is used to hold the mask to the face. The visor lens is made of polycarbonate or other clear, shatterproof, and chemically resistant material. At the bottom of the facepiece is an exhalation value. Some masks include an air-tight speaking diaphragm, which facilitates communications while preventing contaminated air from entering.

SCBA Inspection and Checkout

The SCBA must be inspected according to manufacturer and 29 CFR recommendations. In addition, the SCBA should be checked out immediately prior to use. Checkout and inspection procedures should be followed closely to assure safe operation of the unit.

A cylinder on a SCBA typically carries the following information (FIGURE 3):

- DOT exemption for composite cylinder
- DOT rated pressure and air volume
- Cylinder number
- Manufacturer's name, symbol, and part number
- Original hydrostatic test date, month/year

National Fire Protection Association Standards for SCBAs

The National Fire Protection (NFPA) has developed a standard for performance requirements and appropriate testing procedures designed to simulate various environmental conditions that fire fighter's SCBA can be exposed to during use and storage. These requirements are in addition to the basic NIOSH certification requirements.

- **Basic Design Requirements.** The basic design requirements for SCBA units under are:

  - That the units be NIOSH certified positive-pressure.
  - The maximum weight shall not exceed 35 pounds, in accordance with NIOSH certification.
  - The rated service time shall be 30 minutes or more.
  - No positive-pressure unit that can be switched to demand mode.
  - The unit shall not be approved under the Bureau of Mines Schedule.
  - The manufacturer shall provide with each SCBA instructions on maintenance, storage, disinfecting, inspection, use, operations, limitations, and training materials.

- **General Requirements.** Additionally, SCBA units must meet certain general requirements, which include:
  - Labeling showing that the unit meets the requirements.
  - Initial, annual and fifth year testing of the SCBA.
  - Retesting of unit after any modifications.
  - Test series to include three categories, with one SCBA used per category.
- **Performance Tests: Airflow.** This test increases the current NIOSH breathing machine requirements of 40 liters per minute to 100 liters per minute. The 100 liters per minute volume was derived from a review of several studies indicating that a ventilation rate of 100 standard liters per

minute encompasses the 98th percentile of all fire fighters studies.

NOTE: An airflow test is then performed after each of the following tests, with the exception of the fabric component test, to ensure breathing apparatus performance.

- **Thermal Resistance Test.** This series of tests exposes the breathing apparatus to various temperature extremes and temperature cycles that breathing apparatus might be exposed to during actual firefighting operations.
- **Vibration and Shock.** This test is designed to provide a reasonable level of assurance that when the breathing apparatus is exposed to vibration, such as being carried on a rig that often travels over rough road surfaces, the apparatus will perform and function properly.
- **Fabric Components Test.** Flame, heat, and threat tests are added to provide a reasonable level of assurance that the fabric components of a harness assembly used to hold the backplate to the wearer's body will remain intact during firefighting operations.
- **Accelerated Corrosion Resistance Test.** This test is to provide a reasonable level of assurance that the breathing apparatus is designed to resist corrosion that may form and interfere with the apparatus performance and function.
- **Particulate Resistance Test.** This test exposes the breathing apparatus to a specified concentration of particulates to provide a reasonable level of assurance that the apparatus is designed to properly function when exposed to dust conditions commonly present during firefighting operations.
- **Facepiece Lens Abrasion Resistance Test.** This test is designed to provide a reasonable level of assurance that the facepiece lens of the breathing apparatus is not easily scratched during firefighting operations that could result in reduced visibility for the fire fighter.
- **Communications Test.** This test is designed to assure that the facepiece of the breathing apparatus does not significantly reduce a fire fighter's normal voice communications.

Employee Training, Instruction and Discipline

1. Every employee who is required to wear a respirator must know how to wear it, care for it, adjust it and know how to determine if it fits properly and provides the appropriate protection.

2. Each supervisor will provide their employees with needed respirator training and instruction.

3. Such training and instruction will be given to any employee under the supervisor's direct and immediate control if the employee has not already received it OR if the employee's prior training/instruction did not satisfy OSHA requirements, or if any doubt or question exists about respirator use or of any of the matters mentioned in this program.

4. Additional training (on a daily basis if necessary) will be provided by each supervisor whenever it is needed to protect the health and safety of employees.

5. Each respirator wearer shall be given an opportunity to handle the respirator, have it fitted properly, test its facepiece-to-face seal, wear it in normal air for a period of time long enough to gain familiarity with it, have the respirator fit-tested as required by the applicable OSHA regulation and to wear the respirator in a test atmosphere.

6. Each respirator is accompanied by its own set of instructions for proper use, care and protection as well as its limitations. The instructions are printed in or on the respirator box, bag or container. These instructions must be observed.

7. Each respirator wearer must read and abide by these instructions.

8. Any employee who does not understand the respirator instructions must immediately his/her supervisor for assistance.

9. Any employee who has not been provided with all of the training and instruction set forth above, or at any time is unsure about respirator use, care or protection, or has any problems or difficulties with work while wearing a respirator, must inform his or her supervisor at once so that the employee can be provided with the proper training and instruction.

10. Failure to follow all instructions and training on use, care and protection and/or failure to wear respirator during times of exposure can reduce respirator effectiveness and result in sickness or death. The vapors and mists that can be dangerous to health

include particulates or gasses that may not be visible with the normal eye.

11. It is vital to each employee's health that the respirator training and instruction be observed; AND it is vital to each employee's job.

12. Appropriate discipline will be taken against any employee who fails to observe any portion of the OSU respirator program.

13. Persons who provide respirator training and instruction must make sure a written record is provided of the required training and fit-test.

RESPIRATOR QUALITATIVE FIT TEST FORM

EMPLOYEE INFORMATION	
Employee Name	Date of Test
SSAN	Job Title
Telephone (Business)	(Home)

INFORMATION ON FIT TESTER	
Name:	Signature:
SSAN	Company/Job Title
Telephone (Business)	(Home)

Qualitative Fit Test Selected:	☐ Banana Oil	☐ Solution
Fit Test Problems:	☐ Beard Growth ☐ Facial scaring	☐ Dentures ☐ Prosthetics	☐ Glasses ☐ Cosmetic Surgery

SENSITIVITY TEST

No.	Procedure
1.	Sensitivity test conducted

RESPIRATOR SELECTION

No.	Procedure
1.	Respirator selection conducted in different room as fit testing
2.	Reviewed Respirator donning/fitting techniques with test subject
3.	Assessed comfort of selected mask by reviewing the following: Positioning mask on the nose; Room for eye protection; Room to talk; Positioning mask on face and cheeks
4.	Adequacy of respirator fit: Chin properly placed; Snap tension; Fit across nose bridge; Distance from nose to chin; Tendency to slip; Self-observation in mirror
5.	Test subject selected the most comfortable respirator from a selection of at least two manufacturers and at least five sizes
6.	Test subject conducted negative and positive pressure checks
7.	Test subject questioned again regarding comfort of respirator after passing the fit test (if not comfortable, allow selection of another model)

| 8. | Test subject given the opportunity to select a different facepiece and be retested if respirator becomes uncomfortable at any time during the test |
| 9. | After selecting, donning, and properly adjusting a respirator, the test subject wore it to the fit test room. The subject wore the respirator at least 10 minutes before entering the fit test chamber. Once in the fit test chamber, two minutes passed before beginning the fit test exercises listed below |

FIT TEST	
No.	Test Exercises (length of time for each test is one minute)
1.	Breathe normally.
2.	Breathe deeply. Be certain breaths are deep and regular.
3.	Turn head all the way from one side to the other. Inhale on each side. Be certain movement is complete. Do not bump the respirator against the shoulders.
4.	Nod head up-and-down. Inhale when head is in the full up position. Be certain motions are complete and made about every second. Do not bump the respirator on the chest.
5.	Talking. The following is called the "Rainbow Passage." *Hand a copy of this passage (alternatives can be used) printed on a card and instruct the test subject to read it aloud and slowly:* "When the sunlight strikes raindrops in the air, they act like a prism and form a rainbow. The rainbow is a division of white light into many beautiful colors. These take the shape of a long round arch, with its path high above, and its two ends apparently beyond the horizon. There is, according to legend, a boiling pot of gold at one end. People look but no one ever finds it. When a man looks for something beyond reach, his friends say he is looking for the pot of gold at the end of the rainbow."

FIT TEST PASSAGE	
No.	Criteria for passing/failing fit test
1.	If at any time during the test, the subject detects the solution, the test has failed. If the test has failed, the test subject must return to the respirator selection room , remove the failed respirator, and select a new respirator as described in the respirator selection section of this form. For this test, the respirator:

FIT TEST OPTIONS	
No.	Available options
1.	The fit test cannot be conducted if there is any hair growth between the skin and the facepiece sealing surface. Did the test subject have any hair growth between the skin and facepiece sealing surface?
2.	At least two facepieces must be selected. The test subject must be given the opportunity to wear them for one week to choose the one which is more comfortable to wear. Did test subject need the opportunity to wear two facepieces for a week?
3.	If a person cannot pass the fit test described above wearing a half mask respirator from the available selection, full facepiece models must be used. Did test subject pass the fit test using a half mask respirator?

RESPIRATOR FIT CERTIFICATION

This is to certify that _________________________ has been successfully fit tested and trained in
ASSOCIATE
respirator use and care and is qualified to wear the following respirators:

1. ______________________ __________   2. ______________________ ________
   RESPIRATOR BRAND/TYPE   SIZE   RESPIRATOR BRAND/TYPE   SIZE

3. ______________________ ____ ______   4. ______________________ ________
   RESPIRATOR BRAND/TYPE   SIZE   RESPIRATOR BRAND/TYPE   SIZE

5. ______________________ ______   6. ______________________ ________
   RESPIRATOR BRAND/TYPE   SIZE   RESPIRATOR BRAND/TYPE   SIZE

RESPIRATOR FIT TEST FORM RETENTION INFORMATION

Permanent Retention File:	Location:
Date Filed:	Filed By:

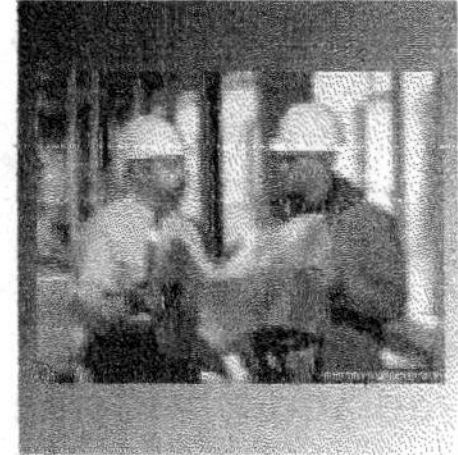

The primary objective when responding to a hazardous material incident is the prevention, or reduction, of detrimental effects to public health or environment. To accomplish this, it is necessary to:

- Identify the substance involved.

- Evaluate its behavior when released and its effects on public health and the environment.

- Initiate actions to prevent or modify its effects.

A high priority, from start to finish of an incident, is obtaining the necessary information to evaluate its impact. This is called incident characterization and is the process of identifying the substance involved and evaluating actual, or potential, impact on public health or the environment.

Characterization is relatively straightforward in incidents where the substance involved is known or easily identified; the pathways of dispersion are clearly defined; and the effect or potential impact is demonstrated. For example, the effects of a large discharge of vinyl chloride on fish in a small stream is relatively easy to evaluate. However, an incident such as an abandoned waste site containing 60,000 fifty-five gallon drums is more complex because there generally is not enough initial information to determine the hazards and to evaluate their impact.

Evaluating a hazardous substance incident is generally a two-phase process: (1) an initial characterization, and (2) a more comprehensive characterization.

Preliminary Assessment

At site responses where the hazards are largely unknown and where there is no need to go on-site immediately, conduct an off-site reconnaissance by: (1) making visual observations; (2) monitoring atmospheric hazards near the site and (3) collecting off-site samples that may indicate on-site conditions or migration from the incident.

An off-site reconnaissance and information gathering should also include:

- Collections of information not available from, or needed to verify or supplement, the preliminary assessment.

- General layout and map of the site.

- Monitoring ambient air with direct-reading instruments for: oxygen deficiency; combustible gases; radiation; organic vapors, gases, particulates; inorganic vapors, gases, particulates; and specific materials if known.

- Placards, labels, markings on containers or transportation vehicles.

- Configuration of containers, tank cars, and trailers.

- Types and number of containers, building, and impoundments.

- Biological indicators – dead vegetation, animals, insects, and fish.

- Unusual odors or conditions.

- Visual observation of vapors, clouds, or suspicious substances.

- Off-site samples (surface water, drinking water, site run-off, groundwater, soil, air).

- Interviews with inhabitants, observers, or witnesses.

Initial characterization

The initial characterization is based on information that is readily available or that can be quickly obtained. This information is used to determine: (1) what hazards exist and (2) if immediate protective measures are necessary. During this initial phase, a number of key decisions must be made as follows:

- Imminent or potential risk to public health and to the environment.

- Immediate need for protective actions to prevent or reduce the impact.

- Protection of the health and safety of response personnel.

Once immediate control measures are implemented, actions can start to restore the area to environmentally acceptable conditions. If there is no emergency, time can be spent to: (1) evaluate hazards; (2) design cleanup plans; and (3) establish safety requirements for response personnel. Also, information to characterize the hazards can be obtained from intelligence (records, placards, eye witnesses, etc.), direct reading instruments, and sampling. Various combinations of these information gathering techniques can be used dependent upon the nature of the incident and the time available.

The outline that follows lists the types of data necessary to evaluate the impact of a hazardous materials incident. Not every incident requires all items to be obtained. However, the list does provide a guide that can be adapted to meet site-specific conditions.

Data Gathering and Preliminary Assessment. Upon notification or discovery of an incident, obtain the following information:

- Brief description.
- Exact location.
- Date and time of occurrence.
- Hazardous materials involved and their physical/chemical properties.
- Present status of incident.
- Potential pathways of dispersion.
- Habitation – population at risk.
- Environmentally sensitive areas – endangered species, delicate ecosystems.
- Economically sensitive areas – industrial, agricultural.
- Accessibility by air and roads.
- Waterways.
- Current weather and forecast.
- Terrain – include topographic map.
- Geology and hydrology – include appropriate maps.
- Aerial photographs.
- Communications.
- Any other related background information.

Information about an incident, especially abandoned waste sites, may also be available from:

- **Other federal agencies.**
- **State and local health or environmental agencies.**
- **Company records.**
- **Court records.**
- **Water departments, sewage districts.**
- **State and local authorities.**

On-Site Survey

A more thorough evaluation of hazards generally requires personnel to enter the defined site. Before going on-site, an entry plan is developed to: (1) address what will be initially accomplished and (2) give the procedures to protect the health and safety of response personnel. On-site inspection and information gathering includes:

- **Monitoring ambient air with direct-reading instruments for: oxygen deficiency, combustible gases, radiation, organic vapors and gases, inorganic vapors and gases, particulates, and specific materials if known.**

- **Types of containers, impoundments, and their storage system: numbers, types, and quantities of material.**

- **Condition of storage systems (such as state of repair or deterioration).**

- **Leaks or discharges from containers, tanks, ponds, vehicles, etc.**

- **Potential pathways of dispersion: air, surface water, ground water, land surface, biological routes.**

- **Placards, labels, markings, identification tags, or indicators of material.**

- **Container configuration, shape of tank cars, or trailers.**

- **Standing water or liquids.**

- **Condition of soil.**

- **Wells, storage containers, drainage ditches, or streams and ponds.**

Comprehensive Characterization

The second phase, comprehensive characterization (which may not be needed in all responses), is a more methodical investigation to enhance, refine, and enlarge the information base obtained during the preliminary inspection. This phase provides more complete information to characterize the hazards associated with an incident. As a continuously operating program, the second phase also reflects environmental changes resulting from response activities.

Available information and information obtained through initial site entries may be sufficient to thoroughly identify and assess the human and environmental effects of an incident. If not, an environmental surveillance program needs to be implemented. Much of the same type of information as collected during the preliminary inspection is needed. However, it may be much more extensive. Instead of one or two ground water samples being collected, an extensive ground water survey may be needed over a long period of time. Results from the preliminary inspection provide a screening mechanism for a more complete environmental surveillance program to determine the extent of contamination. Also, since mitigation and remedial measures may cause changes in the original conditions, a continual surveillance program must be maintained to identify any changes.

Evaluating the hazards associated with an incident involves various degrees of complexity. The release of a single, known chemical compound may represent a relatively simple problem. It becomes progressively more difficult to determine harmful effects as the number of compounds increases. Evaluation of the imminent, or potential hazards, associated with an abandoned waste site, storage tanks, or lagoons holding vast amounts of known, or unknown, chemical substances is far more complex than a single release of an identifiable substance.

The major responsibility of response personnel is the protection of public health and the environment. The effective accomplishment of this goal is dependent upon a thorough characterization of the chemical compounds involved, their dispersion pathways, concentrations in the environment, and deleterious effects. A base of information is developed over the lifetime of the incident to assess the harmful effects and ensure that effective actions are taken to mitigate the release.

HAZMAT incident strategies

Scene survey and safety precautions - resist rushing in and stay clear of all spills, vapors, fumes and smoke. Others cannot be helped until the situation has been fully assesses. Always approach the scene from uphill up wind and up stream when ever possible unless special circumstances apply. Consider using a "rule of thumb" method to determine minimal safety distances for identifying unknown containers. For small events such as a 55 gallon drum or a singular bag stay at a minimum of 150 feet until the container and its contents can be identified, larger events (more than one drum or bag) complexes or incident hidden by structure 500 feet. Any container in which there is a potential for bleve or conflagration 2500 ft. once the material can be identified refer to your emergency response guide book to aid in implementing your next course of action. "Old school rule of thumb" if you put your thumb up to the haz-mat incident and you can still see the materials involved you're to close.

Secure the scene - without entering the immediate hazard area, isolate the area and assure the safety of people and the environment, keep people away from the scene and outside the safety perimeter. Always allow enough room to move and remove your own equipment.

Identify the hazards - placards, container labels, shipping documents and/or knowledgeable persons on the scene are valuable information sources. Evaluate all available information and consult the recommended response guide (NAERG) to reduce immediate risks. New information, provided by the shipper or obtained from another authoritative source, may change some of the emphasis or details found in the response guide. Remember that the guide provides only the most important and worst case scenario information for the initial response in relation to a family or class of dangerous goods. As more material-specific information becomes available, the response should acclimate to the situation.

Assess the situation - consider the following when responding to a haz-mat incident. Is there a fire, a spill or a leak? What are the weather conditions? What is the terrain like? Who/what is at risk: people, property or the environment? What actions should be taken: is evacuation necessary? Is diking necessary? What resources (human and equipment) are required and are readily available? What can be done immediately?

Obtain help - advise your dispatch of the situation and request that they notify responsible agencies and obtain assistance from qualified personnel.

Respond - establish a command post and lines of communication. Rescue casualties where possible and evacuate id necessary. Maintain control of the site. Continually reassess the situation and modify the response accordingly. The first duty is to consider the safety of people in the immediate area, including your own.

Important - does not walk into or touch spilled material. Avoid inhalation of fumes, smoke and vapors, even if no dangerous goods are known to be involved. Do not assume that the gases or vapors are harmless because of lack of smell- odorless gases or vapors may be harmful.

Who to call for assistance - Upon arrival at the scene, a first responder is expected to recognize the presence of dangerous goods, protect oneself and the public, secure the area and call for assistance of trained personnel as soon as conditions permit. The fro must follow the steps outlined your organizations standard operating procedures and/or local emergency response plan for obtaining qualified assistance. The notification sequence and requests for technical information beyond what is available in your emergency response guidebook should occur in the following order.

1. Organization/Agency

 Notify your organization or agency. This will set in motion a series of events based upon the information provided. Actions may range from dispatching additional trained personnel to the scene to activating the local emergency response plan. Ensure that other local fire and police departments have been notified.

2. Emergency Response Telephone Number

Locate and call the telephone number located on the shipping document. The person answering the phone at the listed emergency response number must be knowledgeable of the materials and mitigation actions to be taken, or must have immediate access to a person who has the required knowledge.

3. National Assistance

 Contact the appropriate emergency response agency listed in the back of your emergency response guidebook when the emergency response telephone number is unavailable. Upon receipt of a call describing the nature of the incident, the agency will provide immediate advice on handling the early stages of the incident. The agency will also contact the shipper or manufacturer of the material(s) for more detailed information and request on-scene assistance when necessary.

Collect and provide as much of the following information as can safely be obtained, such as:
- Your name, call back telephone number, fax number
- Location and nature of problem
- Name and identification number of material(s) involved
- Shipper/consignee/point of origin
- Carrier name, rail car or truck
- Container type and size
- Quantity of material(s) transported/released
- Local conditions (weather, terrain, proximity to school & hospitals)
- Injuries and exposures
- Local emergency services that have been notified

4. <u>Special Notes</u>

 1. The appropriate federal agency must be notified in the case of rail, air or marine incidents

2. The nearest police department must be notified in the case of lost stolen or misplaced explosives, radioactive materials or infectious substances.

HAZARDOUS MATERIALS INCIDENT SITE SAFETY PLAN

Incident Name _TRAIN WRECK_ Date _1/6/05_ Operational Period _1/6/05 - 1/8/05_

Site Information

Incident Location _GRANITVILLE, SC_
Safe Access Route _______________________________
Command Post Location _____________________________
Control Zones _HOT - 2000 FT_
 Exclusion _WARM - SMLS_
 Contamination Control _COOL - ABOVE SMLS_
Support ____
Weather Conditions ______________________________
Wind Direction _____________ Speed ____________ Temp/Time __________
Forecast _______________________________________

<u>**Organization**</u>

Incident Commander _______________________________________
Hazmat (HM) Group Supervisor _____________________________
HM Technical Reference ___________________________________
Safe Refuge Area Manager _________________________________
Safety Officer ____
Site Access Control ______________________________________
Entry Leader ____
Decon Leader ____
Entry Team ____
   1. ____
   2. ____
   3. ____
   4. ____
Back Up
   1. ____
   2. ____
   3. ____
   4. ____
Decon
   1. ____
   2. ____
   3. ____
   4. ____

<u>***Hazard Evaluation***</u>

Chemical Names(s) ____
Hazards ____
General Hazards and Safety Precautions ___________________

<u>**Monitoring**</u>

LEL Instruments _4 GAS meter_____   ( ) Continuous or _____
02 Instruments _______   ( ) Continuous or _____
Toxicity/ppm Instruments ______   ( ) Continuous or _____
Radiological Instruments ______   ( ) Alpha ____ Beta ____ _ELECTRON_
                            ( )Gama_____

Helium ATOM

<u>**Protective Clothing**</u>

Entry ____

Decon _____ *I LEVEL LOWER THAN ENTRY TEAM*

<u>**Decontamination**</u>

Decontamination Corridor Location _____ *AWAY FROM WIND*
FROM RED TO COOL
Decon Layout _______________________________________

Decon solution for Personnel _______________________
Decon solution for Equipment _______________________

<u>**Communications**</u>

Radio Frequencies Assigned _________________________
    Command _______________________________________
    Tactical _______________________________________
Cellular Telephone Numbers _________________________

Additional Communications __________________________

<u>**Emergency Procedures**</u>

Safe Refuge Area ___________________________________

Escape/Evacuation Alarm ____________________________

Emergency First Aid Location _______________________

<u>***Plan Review***</u>

Safety Officer Signature ___________________________
                  Time _______ Date _______
HM Group Supervisor Signature ______________________
                  Time _______ Date _______
Incident Commander Signature _______________________
                  Time _______ Date _______

Incident Name _____________________ Date _______
Operational Period _______________

<u>**Plan Amendment**</u>
Check Amended Section:
- ❑ Site Information
- ❑ Organization
- ❑ Hazard Evaluation
- ❑ Monitoring
- ❑ Protective Clothing
- ❑ Decontamination
- ❑ Emergency Procedures
- ❑ Plan Review

Amended Information
<u>Plan Review</u>
Safety Officer Signature _________________________________Time________
Date________

HM Group Supervisor Signature
___________________________ Time ________ Date ________

Incident Commander Signature
___________________________ Time ________ Date________

<u>CHEMICAL INFORMATION SHEET</u>

DOT Placard _______________

<u>Common Name</u> ___________
Chemical Name ____________
Chemical Formula __________

Physical Description ____
Liquid __________ Solid _________ Gas __________
Chemical Structure ________________________________
Vapor Density ___________________________________
Specific Gravity __________________________________
Flash Point ______________________________________
Flammable Range _________________________________
Solubility _______________________________________
Boiling Point ____________________________________
Melting Point ____________________________________
Vapor Pressure __________________________________
Other ____
Incompatibilities _________________________________

PRIMARY HEALTH HAZARDS:
Concentrations
(PEL, TLV, other)

Ingestion ____

Skin/eye absorption _______________________________________

Skin/eye contact____

Carcinogen ____

Teratogen ____

Mutagen ____

Combustibility____

Toxic by-products ____

Flammability____

Explosivity ____

LEL____

Uel ____

Reactivities ____

Corrosivity ____

pH____

Neutralizing Agent ____

Recommended PPE: _______________________________________

Sources of Technical Information:

Chapter 6 -DECONTAMINATION

There are a number of ways that hazardous waste site workers and emergency responders may become contaminated such as:

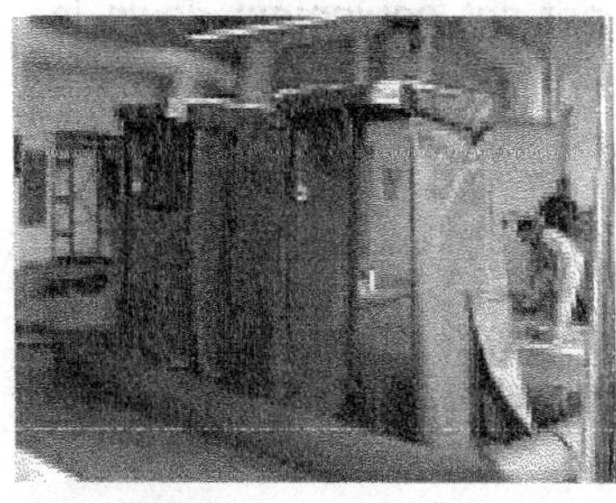

- Contact with gases, mists, vapors, or particulates in the air.

- Splash from materials while sampling or working.

- Walking, sitting, touching, or handling contaminated liquids, soils, or equipment.

Protective clothing and respirators help prevent the worker from coming in contact with contaminants, while proper work practices help to reduce the contact and spread of contaminants. Care must be taken to prevent the transfer of contaminants to clean areas and to prevent exposing unprotected personnel. In order to prevent such events, contamination reduction and decontamination procedures must be developed and implemented as part of the health and safety plan before any activity begins. These procedures should include: the number of decontamination stations, equipment needed, methods to minimize overall contamination, and disposal methods.

Decontamination has four primary goals:

- To protect workers from hazardous substances that may contaminate and eventually permeate the protective clothing, respiratory equipment, tools, and vehicles used on-site.

- To protect all site personnel by reducing/minimizing the transfer of contaminants to clean areas.

- To prevent the mixing/contact of incompatible substances.

- To protect the community from the migration of contaminants off-site.

<u>**Initial Planning**</u>

Some considerations must be given when developing a decontamination plan:

- Stress work practices that minimize contact with contaminants (e.g., do not work in puddles, do not set equipment down in obvious contamination).

- Use remote sampling, handling, and container opening techniques.

- Protect monitoring and sampling instruments by bagging (making openings in the bags for sample ports, probes, sensors, etc.)

- Wear disposable outer garments and use disposable equipment where appropriate.

- Cover equipment and tools with strippable coating which can be removed during decontamination.

- Encase the source of contaminants (e.g., plastic or overpacks).

- Use protective liner when setting equipment on the ground.

<u>**Zone Layout**</u>

An area within the **Contamination Reduction Zone**, or CRZ, is designated as the **Contamination Reduction Corridor**, or CRC. The CRC controls access into and out of the **Exclusion Zone** and confines personnel decontamination activities to a limited area. The size of the corridor depends on the number of stations in the decontamination procedure, the overall dimensions of work control zones, and the amount of space available. A corridor or 75 X 15 feet should be adequate for full decontamination. Whenever possible, it should be a straight path.

The CRC boundaries should be conspicuously marked with entry and exit restricted. The far end is the **hotline**, the boundary between the Exclusion Zone and the Contamination Reduction Zone. Personnel exiting the Exclusion Zone must go through the CRC. Anyone in the CRC should be wearing the level of protection designated for the decontamination crew. Another corridor may be required for the entrance and exit of heavy equipment needing decontamination. Within the CRC, distinct areas are set aside for the decontamination of personnel, portable field equipment, removed clothing, etc. These areas should be marked and restricted to those personnel wearing the appropriate level of protection. All activities within the corridor are confined to decontamination.

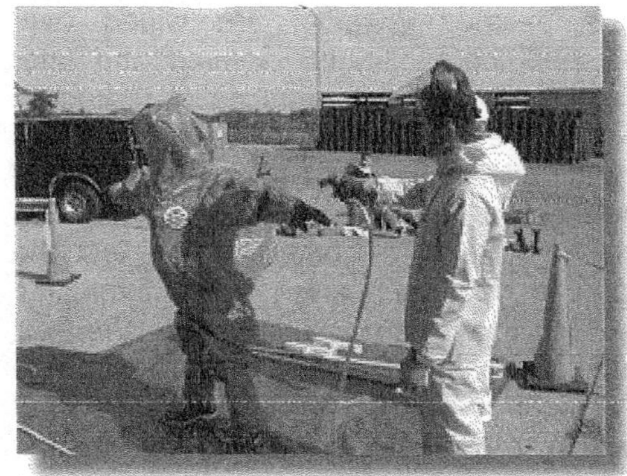

Protective clothing, respirators, monitoring equipment, sampling supplies, and other equipment are all maintained outside the CRC. Personnel don their protective equipment away from the CRC and enter the Exclusion Zone through a separate access control point at the hotline.

FIGURE 1
CONTAMINATION REDUCTION ZONE LAYOUT

Decontamination Worker Protection

Generally, decontamination workers will either don the same level of protection that is worn by workers in the Exclusion Zone or downgrade one level of protection. In any case, the level of protection for decontamination workers is relative to the site in question and the worker's position in the decontamination line.

The level of protection worn by decontamination workers is determined by:

- Expected or visible contamination on workers.
- Type(s) of contaminant(s) and associated respiratory and skin hazards.
- Total vapor/gas concentrations in the CRC.
- Particulates and specific inorganic or organic vapors in the CRC.
- Results of swipe tests.
- The presence (or suspected presence) of highly toxic or skin-destructive materials.

Effectiveness of Decontamination

There is no method of determining immediately how effective decontamination is in removing contaminants. Discolorations, stains, corrosion, and residues on objects may indicate that contaminants have not been removed. However, observable effects only indicate surface contamination and not permeation (absorption) into clothing. Many contaminants are not easily observed.

One method for determining the effectiveness of surface decontamination is **swipe testing**. Cloth or paper patches (swipes) are wiped over predetermined surfaces of the suspect contaminated clothing and later analyzed in a laboratory. Both the inner and outer surfaces of protective clothing should be swipe tested. Positive results for both sets of swipes would indicate that surface contamination has not been removed and substances have penetrated or permeated the garment. Swipe tests can also be performed on skin or inside clothing. Another way to test the effectiveness of decontamination procedures is to analyze the contaminants left in the cleaning solutions. Elevated levels of contaminants in the final rinse solution may suggest that additional cleaning and rinsing are needed. As noted, laboratory analysis is required for the aforementioned test methods. As can be seen, lab testing provides after-the-fact information. However, along with visual observations, results of these tests can help in ascertaining the effectiveness of decontamination. In addition, the decision-making chart can aid in evaluating the health and safety aspects of decontamination methods

Decontamination Solutions

Protective equipment, sampling tools, and other equipment are usually decontaminated by scrubbing with detergent water using a soft-bristle brush, followed by rinsing with copious amounts of water. While this process may not be fully effective in removing some contaminants (in some cases, the contaminants may react with water), it is a relatively safe option compared to the use of other decontamination solutions. The contaminant must be identified before a decontamination chemical is used, and reactions of such a chemical with unidentified substances or mixtures and personal protective equipment could be especially troublesome. A decontamination solution must always be selected in consultation with an experienced chemist and an industrial hygienist. Although it is recommended that water be used for decontamination as much as possible,

Disposal of Contaminated Materials

All materials and equipment used for decontamination must be disposed of properly. Clothing, tools, buckets, brushes, and all other equipment that are contaminated must be secured in drums or other containers and labeled. Clothing not completely contaminated on the site should be secured in plastic bags pending further decontamination and/or disposal.

Contaminated wash and rinse solutions can be kept temporarily in a step-in container (for example, a child's wading pool) or in a plastic-lined trench about four inches deep. Such solutions are ultimately transferred to labeled drums and disposed of with other substances on the site. Generally, hazardous waste or industrial haulers are called upon to handle the ultimate disposal of decontamination equipment and drums.

Medical Emergency Decontamination

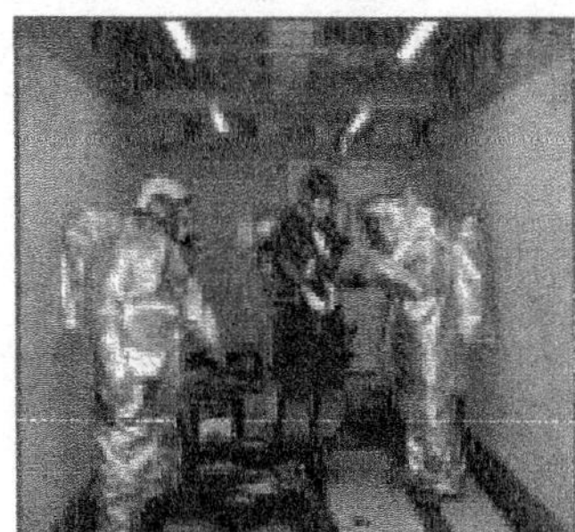

When outlining decontamination procedures in the health and safety plan, provisions must be made for decontaminating personnel with medical problems and injuries. There is the possibility that decontamination may aggravate a health problem or cause more serious problems. For example, lifesaving care should be instituted immediately without considering decontamination. The outside garments can be removed (depending on the weather) if this does not cause delays, interfere with treatment, or aggravate the problem. Respiratory masks and backpack assemblies must always be removed. Fully encapsulating suits or chemical-resistant clothing can be cut away. If the outer contaminated garments cannot be safely removed, the individual should be wrapped in plastic, rubber, or blankets to help prevent contaminating medical personnel and/or the inside of ambulances. Outside garments are then removed at the medical facility. Whenever possible, response personnel should accompany contaminated victims to the medical facility to advise on matters involving decontamination. No attempt should be made to wash or rinse the victim unless it is known that the victim has been contaminated with an extremely toxic or corrosive material that could also cause severe injury or loss of life. For minor medical problems or injuries, the normal decontamination procedures should be followed.

RADIATION

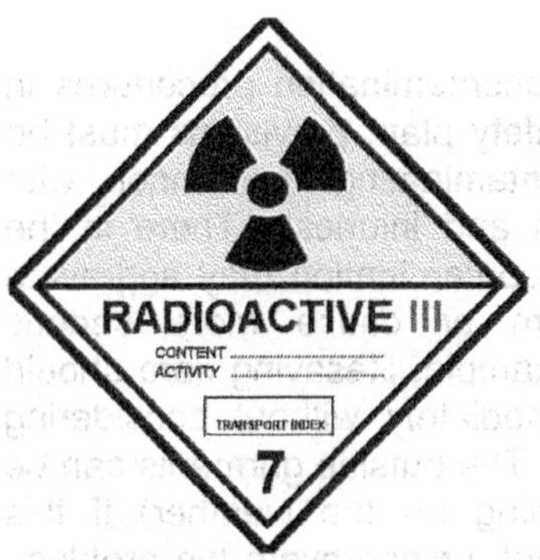

There are three primary categories of radiation that might be encountered in a field survey: (1) alpha; (2) beta; and (3) gamma. Each of these has unique properties that must be considered in selecting an instrument for use. Alpha particles are simply energetic helium ions, i.e., atoms that have lost their electrons. Because of their large size (compared to other forms of radiation) and high charge, they will not penetrate through much matter. They will penetrate through more material than alphas, but generally can be stopped by a thin piece of metal. Gamma radiation is simply high energy light and is the most penetrating of the radiation types. Very high energy gammas can penetrate through several centimeters of lead.

There are hazards associated with exposure of humans to radiation, but if the exposure is limited to low levels, that hazard is not very serious. In fact, humans are exposed to natural background radiation every day. Naturally occurring radioactive materials can be found in the soil, building materials, certain foods, and even the human body. The unit used to quantify the radiation dose received by an individual is the roentgen equivalent man (REM). The average dose, due to natural background radiation and natural radioactive materials in the environment, to an individual in the United States is about 0.2 rem/year.

The actual health risk from low levels of radiation is quite small. There is no direct evidence that low doses to radiation can injure the health of humans. All of the estimates of the health risks associated with radiation have been extrapolated from studies of people who have received doses equivalent to hundreds of rem. It has been assumed that very low levels of radiation would affect the body in the same way as these very high doses, only with proportionately less damage. As radiation passes through matter, it may interact and lose energy. The damage done by radiation as it interacts with the body results from the way it affects molecules essential to the normal functioning of human cells. One of four things may happen when radiation strikes a cell: (1) the radiation may pass through the cell without doing any damage; (2) the cell may be damaged but repairs itself; (3) the cell may be damaged so that it not only fails to repair itself, but reproduces in damaged form over a period of years; or (4) the cell may be killed. The death of a single cell may not be harmful since the body can readily replace most cells, but problems will occur if so many cells are killed that the body cannot properly function. Incompletely or imperfectly repaired cells can lead to delayed health effects such as cancer genetic mutations, or birth defects. Again, it is important to recognize that the risks from radiation are small. For example, the statistical risk of a cancer death from 7 millirem of radiation is equivalent to that associated with smoking a single cigarette.

Radiation cannot be detected by any of the human senses. We cannot taste, smell, feel, see, or hear it. Because of this, we must rely upon instruments that respond to an interaction between the radiation and the instrument itself. Radiation is nothing more than energetic particles or photons.

As the radiation passes through matter, it interacts with the material's electrons to lose some of the energy. This energy results in either excitation or ionization of atoms. Depending upon the type of detector, either the excitation or the ionization is sensed, quantified, and the instrument produces a response that is proportional to the total amount of radiation that is present in the area being monitored or surveyed.

Portable survey instruments are calibrated to read out in either counts per minute (CPM), in direct units or radiation intensity, such as milli-roenten/hour (mR/hr) or micro-roentgen/hour (µR/hr). Instruments reading out in mR/hr and µR/hr are used to measure extended radiation fields such as that experienced in the vicinity of radioactive materials storage or disposal sites. Instruments that read out in CPM are usually used to monitor for low-level surface contamination, particularly on hard, non-porous surfaces.

One of the difficulties in measuring radiation is that there is always some background level of radiation present. This background will vary with location; some regions of the country will have higher background than others, brick buildings will have higher backgrounds than wooden buildings, etc. Because of this variation, when any survey instrument is used, a determination of local background must be made in an area that is not believed to contain any radioactive materials. Any reading significantly above the background (two to three times background) is indicative of the presence of radioactive materials. Background levels throughout the United States will typically range between 5 and 100 µR/hr. The United States Environmental Protection Agency (EPA) limits the radiation exposure to workers to 1mR/hr above background. This action level is contained in the EPA's Standard Operation Safety Guides.

The detectors used in most portable survey instruments are gas-filled or scintillation devices. The gas-filled detectors measure the amount of ionization in the gas that is caused by radiation entering the detectors. This is accomplished by establishing a voltage potential across a volume of gas. When the gas is ionized, the current that flows between the electrodes producing the potential can be measured. The amount of current is directly proportional to the amount of radiation that enters the detector. Scintillation detectors depend upon light that is produced in a crystal plastic, of certain compounds, when the material's atoms are excited by interactions with radiation. The amount of light produced is measured and converted to an easily monitored electrical signal by a photomultiplier tube. There are gas-filled and scintillation detectors designed to detect all three of the radiation types of interest in field surveys.

The most obvious difference in detectors used for different radiation types is the manner in which radiation can enter the sensitive volume of the detector. Many gamma survey instruments will not appear to have a detector, but only an electronics box. This is because the gammas can easily penetrate the metal electronics enclosure and the detector is placed inside where it is protected from damage. The Ludlum Model 19 Micro R meter is an example of such a detector. Alpha and beta detectors must have thin entrance windows so that these particles can enter the sensitive volume. Some gas filled detectors are designed with a thick metal shield so they can discriminate between betas and gammas; with the shield open, the detector is sensitive to both betas and gammas; with it closed, it will detect only gammas, since the shield absorbs the betas before they can interact with the detector.

A good survey meter should be portable, rugged, sensitive, simple in construction, and reliable. Portability implies lightness and compactness with a suitable handle or strap for carrying. Ruggedness requires that an instrument be capable of withstanding mild shock without damage. Sensitivity demands an instrument that will respond to the type of energy level of the radiation being measured. Rarely does one find an instrument capable of measuring all types of energies of radiation that are encountered in practice. Simplicity in construction necessitates convenient arrangement of components and simple circuitry comprised of parts that may be replaced easily. Reliability is that attribute that implies ability to duplicate response under similar circumstances.

Ludlum Model 19 Micro R Meter

The Ludlum Model 19 Micro R Meter is designed to monitor low-level gamma radiation. The instrument utilizes an internally mounted sodium iodide scintillator crystal. The meter face has two scales, one in black representing 0-50 μR/hr and one in red representing 0-25 μR/hr. The meter range is controlled with a six position switch: OFF, 5000, 500, 250, 50, and 25. The full-scale reading of the meter is equal to the switch setting; the red scale corresponds to the 25 and 250 position and the black scale to the other three positions. As an example, if the switch is in the 500 position and the meter pointer is aligned with the "30" scale marking, the radiation field is 300 μR/hr.

The Ludlum Model 19 is equipped with five additional switches or buttons. One button, labeled L, lights the meter face while depressed. This allows accurate readings in poor lighting conditions. The BAT button tests the battery condition. If the batteries are good, the meter pointer will deflect to the "batt OK" portion of the scale. The audio switch controls the audible signal; in the ON position, a "beeping" signal accompanies each radiation event that is detected. The switch marked with the F and S controls the meter response; the S (slow) position is used for most applications, although in conditions where the radiation level is changing rapidly, the F (fast) position will provide a better representation of the radiation level. The remaining button resets the detector operating high voltage should a transient pulse cause it to be disabled.

Detector Probes

Detector probes will fall into two major categories: gas-filled detectors and scintillation detectors. These have been briefly discussed in the introduction section. This section will describe a few of the most commonly used probes.

The Geiger-Mueller (GM) pancake probe is very common and is most valuable for monitoring for surface activity on equipment, benchtops, soil surface, and personnel. The probe may be used to monitor alpha, beta, or gamma radiation. The sensitive volume of the detector is covered with a thin mica window of about 1.75 inch diameter. This window allows detection of alphas and low energy betas. The fragile window is protected by a metal screen, and care must be taken to avoid puncturing it.

End-window GM probes may also be used for alpha, beta, and gamma monitoring. These tubes are generally cylindrical, about 6-8 inches long and have mica entrance windows about 1 inch in diameter. The window often does not have a protective screen and is easily punctured. Because of its configuration, this tube is not as convenient as a pancake probe for surface monitoring. Also, because of the smaller entrance window, it is less efficient for detecting alphas and betas.

Thin walled GM probes are used for beta and gamma detection. The tube is constructed within steel walls through which betas can pass. The tube is housed in a protective cage fitted with a moveable steel shield. With the shield in place, betas are absorbed and only gammas can be detected. When the shield is moved away from the cage opening, the detector is sensitive to both betas and gammas.

Scintillation probes are available for alphas, betas, and gammas. They differ in the type of scintillator used and the detector housing. Alpha detectors are made of thin activated zinc sulfide crystals. The beta detectors generally use thin scintillation plastic crystals. Gamma probes use thick crystals of activated sodium iodide. Beta and alpha probes have entrance windows of thin aluminized mylar. This window protects the detector from light which would be sensed by the photomultiplier as if it were a high radiation field. Care must be taken not to puncture the window.

The alpha probes often have large surface areas (50-100 cm^2) to allow efficient detection of low levels of alpha contamination. The gamma detectors are usually housed in an aluminum shell. This shell is not easy to puncture and is quite rugged, although dropping or banging it against a hard object may break the crystal or the photomultiplier.

Personnel Dosimeters

The amount of radiation dose received by an individual working in a radiation field is measured by the use of personnel dosimeters. Two types that are frequently used are the direct reading dosimeter and the thermoluminescent dosimeter (TLD).

The direct reading dosimeter provides an immediate indication of the gamma radiation dose the wearer has received. By checking his dosimeter periodically, the wearer can get an up-to-the-minute estimate of the total gamma dose he/she has received. Only gamma radiation is measured. There is no way that beta radiation can penetrate the walls of the dosimeter to cause ionization.

Inside the detection chamber of the dosimeter is a stationary metal electrode with a movable quartz fiber attached to it. The dosimeter is charged so that both the electrode and the fiber are positively charged. Since both are positively charged, they repel each other, and the movable fiber moves as far away from the electrode as it can. When gamma radiation causes ionization in the detection chamber, the negative ions move to the positively charged electrode or fiber. The action reduces the positive charge and allows the fiber to move a little closer to the stationary electrode. The movement of the fiber, then, is a measure of the amount of gamma radiation absorbed by the detector.

In direct reading pocket dosimeters, a scale is placed so that the hairline on the scale is the movable fiber. As the fiber moves, the scale indicates the total amount of gamma radiation absorbed by the dosimeter. A magnifying glass inside the dosimeter enables the scale to be read. This provides an immediate estimate of an individual's total gamma exposure.

Anyone who is instructed to wear a direct reading dosimeter should make sure that it is properly charged. When a dosimeter is properly charged, there is sufficient potential between the electrode and the fiber that the fiber is significantly displaced and the hairline on the scale reads near zero. In general, a dosimeter is considered to be adequately charged if it reads below 10mR.

If a dosimeter is not properly charged, a charger must be used to charge it before it can be worn. The dosimeter is pushed into the charger, and the charger control is turned until the dosimeter is zeroed. The dosimeter must be checked again after it is taken out of the charger. Sometimes the hairline shifts when the dosimeter is removed from the charger, and the dosimeter will have to be readjusted so that the hairline will end up at or near zero.

Since the direct reading dosimeter measures the whole-body gamma radiation dose, it should be worn in the major trunk area. When using a dosimeter, care must be taken not to bang or drop it. Rough treatment may cause the electrode to discharge completely, sending the hairline all the way upscale.

Thermoluminescent dosimeters (TLDs) are often used for beta and gamma whole-body measurements. Inside the TLD is a very small quantity of crystalline material called a detector chip that is used to measure beta and gamma exposure. A typical detector chip is approximately 1/8 inch across and 1/32 inch thick.

To understand how a detector chip measures radiation, we first need to go through a short review of electron energy levels. As we know, electrons in a solid material prefer to be in their ground energy state. This is especially true for a crystalline material. If radiation imparts enough energy to one of these electrons, the electron will jump up to a higher, instable energy level. However, since the electron prefers to be in the ground state, it will drop to the ground state and emit the extra energy in the form of heat, x-rays, or light.

In TLD material, there is an in-between state called a metastable state, which acts as an electron trap. When radiation strikes the ground state electron, the electron jumps up and is trapped in the metastable state. It remains there until it gets enough energy to move it up to the unstable state. This energy is supplied when the TLD chip is heated to a high enough temperature. Then the electron will drop back down to the ground state, and, because the TLD chip is a luminiscent material, it will release its extra energy in the form of light. The total quantity of light emitted by electrons returning to the ground state is proportional to the number of electrons that were trapped in the metastable state. The number of electrons trapped in the metastable state is proportional to the amount of beta and gamma radiation that interacts with the material. This means the amount of light emitted when the TLD is heated is proportional to the total amount of beta and gamma radiation interacting with the material.

In the photomultiplier tube, electrons are produced in the photocathode, multiplied across the dynodes, and finally collected on the anode. This then produces a pulse in the circuit that is proportional to the total amount of beta and gamma radiation absorbed by the TLD material.

There are several reasons for using TLDs instead of film badges. One reason is size – TLD chips are so small that they can be taped to the fingers to measure exposure to the extremities without interfering with work. A second reason is sensitivity. The TLD is generally more sensitive than a film badge, more accurate in the low mR range, and able to provide a better overall indication of the total beta/gamma dose received. A third reason is that the TLD chip can be reused after it is read.

As with the direct reading dosimeter, TLD is normally worn in the major body region to give the best indication of whole-body dose. There are times, however, when these devices might be worn on other parts of the body. For example, a TLD might be moved to an arm or a leg if these portions of the body might receive more radiation than the trunk area. An additional device such as a finger ring might also be used to measure an extremity dose. A finger ring contains a TLD chip to measure absorbed dose from beta and gamma radiation.

Chapter 8- RESPONSE ORGANIZATION

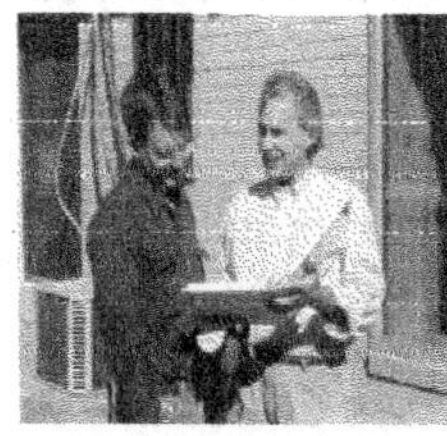

The number of people needed to respond to an incident involving the release or potential release of hazardous substances can vary greatly. To successfully accomplish the primary response goal, of protecting public health and the environment, requires the coordinated, cooperative effort of these people.

Every incident is unique. The hazardous materials involved, their impact on public health and the environment, and the activities required to remedy the event are incident specific. Each incident tends to establish its own operational and organizational requirements. However, common to all incidents are planning, organizational considerations, personnel, and the implementation of operations.

Hazardous Materials Contingency Plans

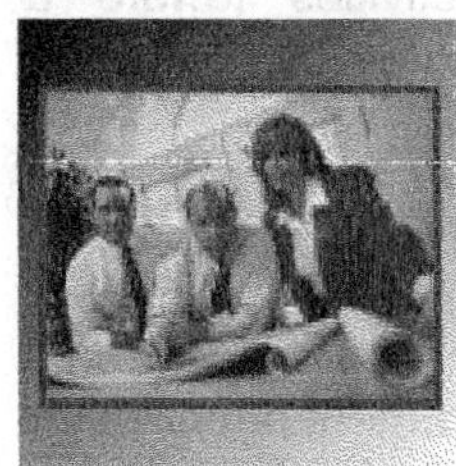

Many of the problems encountered by responders can be reduced if a hazardous materials **contingency plan** exists. When an incident (involving chemicals or other kinds of manmade or natural disasters) occurs, local government reacts. An organization, comprised of all whom are available, will naturally evolve. Its capability, however, to efficiently manage the situation may be severely restricted. Expertise, equipment, and funds needed to prevent or reduce the impact of the event may not be readily available. Necessary actions to ameliorate the situation may be delayed.

A more effective response occurs when a contingency plan exists. In general, contingency plans anticipate the myriad of problems faced by responders and through the planning process solves them. A response organization is established, resources are identified, and prior arrangements made to obtain assistance. A good plan minimizes the delays frequently encountered in a no-plan response, thus permitting more prompt remedial actions. It also reduces the risk to the health of both the responders and public by establishing, in advance, procedures for protecting their safety.

A contingency plan can lessen many of the problems encountered in a response. However, even a good plan cannot anticipate and address all the circumstances created by a release of chemicals. Even with a plan, modifications may be needed in the response organization to accommodate unforeseen situations. A well-written plan acknowledges that adaptations are necessary and provides the framework for doing so without impeding the progress of implementation.

Without a plan, the ability to effectively manage the incident is diminished. Time is wasted attempting to define the problem, get organized, locate resources, and implement response activities. These organizational difficulties can cause delays in the response actions, thus creating additional problems that prompt action would have avoided. For hazardous materials contingency plans to be effective they must be: well-written, agreed upon by all involved, current, flexible, reviewed, and modified and tested.

Organization

The responders needed for an incident may range from a few to hundreds. They represent many government agencies and private industries. Functions and responsibilities of each responders group differ. These diverse elements must be organized into a cohesive unit capable of managing and directing response activities toward a successful conclusion (**FIGURE 1**).

Relatively few well-trained response teams exist. Most response teams are associated with metropolitan fire services or with industry, but are small and may have limited capability or responsibility. In an incident of any magnitude, where more personnel and resources are needed, a team is assembled from the various responding government agencies or private contractors. An organization is then established according to an existing contingency plan. Without a plan, an ad hoc organization is created to manage that specific incident.

The contingency plan or ad hoc organization established, to function effectively must:

- Designate a leader

- Determine objectives

- Establish authority

- Develop policies and procedures

- Assign responsibilities

- Plan and direct operations

- Establish internal communications

- Manage resources (money, equipment, and personnel)

- Establish external communications

In any incident involving more than a few responders, it is generally necessary to develop an organizational chart. This chart depicts the organization's structure. It links personnel and functions, defines lines of responsibility, and establishes internal communication channels. To a large degree, the form and complexity of the organizational chart depends on the magnitude of the incident, the activities needed, the number of people and agencies involved, and the project leader's mode of operation. The key requirements are:

- Establish a chain of command

- Assign responsibilities and functions

- Develop personnel requirements

- Establish internal communications

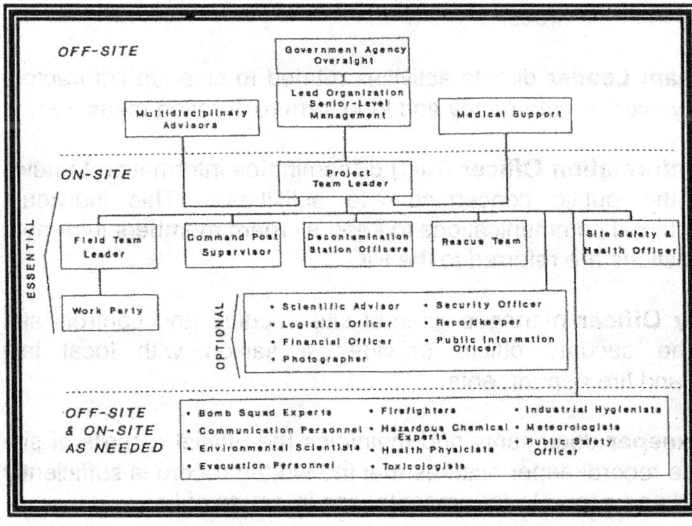

Personnel

To manage and direct the various operations, personnel or responding agencies must be assigned the responsibility for certain activities. The positions, functions, and responsibilities that follow represent personnel requirements for a major response effort. They should be tailored to fit a particular chemical incident. A person must not be assigned responsibility for more than one function.

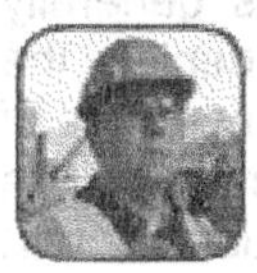

The **Project Leader/On-Scene Coordinator/Incident Manager** (required under 29 CFR 1910.120) has clearly defined authority and responsibility to manage and direct all response personnel and operations while ensuring protection of the health and safety of site personnel and the public.

The **Safety Officer** (required under 29 CFR 1910.120) advises the project leader on all matters related to the health and safety of those involved in site operations. This individual establishes and directs the safety program and coordinates these activities with the scientific advisor. The Safety Officer can halt operations if unsafe conditions exist.

The **Scientific Advisor** directs, coordinates and prioritizes scientific studies, sample collection, field monitoring, analysis of samples, and the interpretation of results. The science advisor may also recommend remedial plans and/or actions and may provide technical guidance to the project leader in those areas.

The **Field Team Leader** directs activities related to cleanup contractors and others involved in emergency and long term restoration measures.

The **Public Information Officer** (PIO) disseminates information to news media and the public concerning site activities. This individual establishes internal communications to keep all team members informed. All media questions are referred to the PIO.

The **Security Officer** manages general site security and controls site access. The security officer provides a liaison with local law enforcement and fire departments.

The **Recordkeeper** documents and maintains the official records of site activities. The recordkeeper assures that the written record is sufficiently clear, detailed and accurate for presentations in courts of law.

The **Field/Operations Officer** directs the activities of team leaders. This individual coordinates these operations with the scientific advisor and safety officer.

The **Team Leaders** manage specific assigned tasks such as: entry team(s), decontamination, sampling teams, monitoring, equipment, photography, and communications.

The **Financial Officer** provides financial and contractual support.

The **Logistics Officer** provides necessary equipment and other resources.

The **Medical Officer** provides medical support and acts as liaison with the medical community.

Implementing Response Operations

The release or potential release of hazardous materials requires operations (or activities) that will eventually restore the situation to normal, or as near as possible to pre-incident conditions. Although each incident establishes its own operational requirements, there is a general sequence of events for all responses. Planning and implementing a response involves, as a minimum, the following:

- **Organize**: Select key personnel. Establish an organization. Assign responsibilities. Modify operations as needed. Institute emergency actions.

- **Evaluate situation**: Based on available information, make preliminary hazard evaluation.

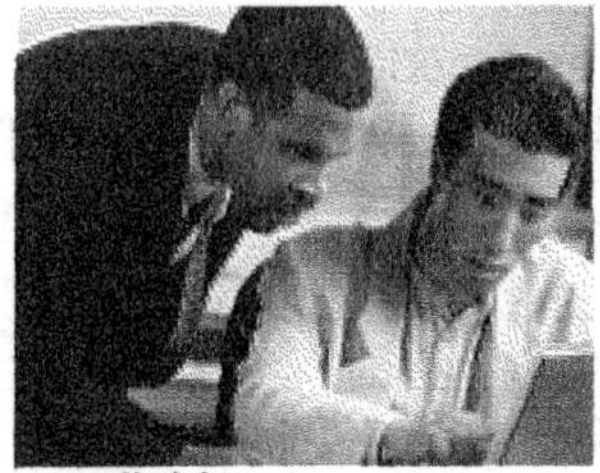

Develop plan of action: Develop preliminary operations plan for gathering and disseminating information; taking immediate counter measures; and implementing emergency and remedial actions. Reevaluate the situation as supplemental information becomes available.

  - Make preliminary off-site survey. Collect additional data to evaluate situation (monitor using direct-reading instruments, sample, make visual observations). Establish emergency actions to protect public health and environment. Identify requirements for on-site reconnaissance. Determine Level of Protection, if necessary, for off-site personnel. Establish boundaries for contaminated areas.

  - Make initial on-site reconnaissance. Collect data (monitor, sample, make visual observations) to determine or verify hazardous conditions and make an overall assessment of the incident. Modify initial entry safety procedures as more data is obtained. Determine levels of protection for initial entry team(s) and subsequent operations. Plan and implement site control and decontamination procedures.

- **Modify original plan of action**: Modify or adapt original plan based on additional information obtained during initial entries. Revise immediate emergency measures. Plan long-term actions including:

  - Additional monitoring and sampling
  - Resource requirements
  - Site safety plan
  - Cleanup and restoration measures
  - Legal implications and litigation
  - Site activity documentation

- **Complete planned cleanup and restoration**

Personnel and Site Reconnaissance

The greatest risk to the safety of responders occurs close to the release. The health and safety of those responders is of paramount importance. Therefore, projected on-site operations must be carefully thought out, well-planned and properly executed. To accomplish this, a site reconnaissance must be completed prior to entering the hazardous substance release area. During this reconnaissance it is necessary to collect as much information as possible in the time available, on the types and hazards, as well as risks that may exist. This information can be obtained from shipping manifests, transportation placards, existing records, container labels, sampling results, monitoring data, or off-site studies.

The Project Leader, after review of intelligence gained from site reconnaissance, makes decisions on the matters that follow:

- Off-site measurements needed

- The need to go on-site

- Equipment available versus equipment needed

- Type of data needed to evaluate hazards such as: organic vapors/gases, inorganic vapors/gases, particulates, oxygen concentration, radiation

- Samples needed for laboratory analysis

- Levels of protection needed by entry team(s)

- Number and size of entry team(s) needed

- Briefing/Debriefing of response team

- Site control procedures which include: designation of work zones, access control, and physical barriers

- Decontamination procedures required

- Medical backup resources available versus needed

- Emergency actions/countermeasures to be taken

- Priority for collecting data and samples

To effectively prevent or reduce the impact of a hazardous materials incident on people or the environment, the personnel responding must be organized into a structured operating unit – a response organization. For the response organization to be effective, it must be developed in advance, be tested, and be an integral part of a Hazardous Materials Contingency Plan. To a large degree, the success of the response is dependent upon how well the response personnel are organized. The more organized, the more rapidly the organization can begin to function. A response organization, once established (whether specified in a contingency plan or as an "ad hoc" incident-specific group) must be flexible enough to adapt to the ever changing conditions created as the incident progresses.

EXAMPLE LIST OF RESPONSE EQUIPMENT

COMMUNICATION EQUIPMENT	**FIELD EQUIPMENT**
Hand-held radios	Combustible gas indicator
	HNU Photoionizer
PROTECTIVE CLOTHING	Organic Vapor Analyzer (OVA)
Fully-Encapsulating Suit	Oxygen meters
Chemical-resistant splash suit	Colorimetric indicator pump/tubes
Chemical-resistant safety boots	Specific gas detectors
Work gloves	Radiation detector
Rain suit	Metal detector
Windbreaker	Pressure-demand SCBAs
Medium weight jacket	Extra air cylinders
Coveralls (work)	Full-face APR (w/canisters)
Coveralls (Nomex)	Photographic equipment
Uniform pants & shirts	Film badges
Socks (regular)	Dosimeters
Socks (heavy)	Organic vapor badges
Underclothes	Hand tool kit (Schedule A)
Earplugs	First Aid kit (Schedule B)
Clipboard	Reference materials (Schedule C)

Hardhat (w/faceshield)	Field support kit (Schedule D)
Hardhat for cold weather	Soil sample set (Schedule E)
Safety goggles	Water sample set (Schedule F)
Safety glasses	Air sample set (Schedule G)
	Emergency oxygen inhaler
	Portable wash unit
	Fire extinguisher
	Portable eyewash

SCHEDULE A: HAND TOOL KIT

Wood mallet	Rubber mallet	Ballpeen hammer
Claw hammer	Hand hammer (non-sparking)	Hacksaw
Lumberjack knife	Duckbill snip	Rod & bolt cutter
Cutting pliers	Lineman's pliers	Slipjoint pliers
Plier wrench	Pipe wrench	Screwdrivers
Stapler/staples	Pressure gauge	Measure tape
Reel tape	Electrical tape	Strapping tape
Duct tape		

SCHEDULE B: FIRST AID KIT

First Aid Guide	Scissors	Aspirin
Forceps	Pain aid	Tweezers
Cold tablets	Cotton swabs	Lozenges
Alcohol swabs	Antiseptic swabs	Antacid
Antiseptic spray	Burn spray	Syrup of ipecac
Spray-on bandage	Vaseline	Eye drops
Antibiotic ointment	Eye/skin neutralizer	Inspect repellent
Eye wash	Sting relief	Adhesive tape
Chigger/tick remover	Cohesive tape	Poison ivy treatment
Snake bite kit	Band-Aids	Ammonia inhalants
Blood clotter	Finger tip bandages	Tourniquet
Knuckle bandages	Ice packs	Elastic strip bandages
Triangle bandages	Salt tablets	Gauze bandages
Finger splint	Blanket	Stretcher

SCHEDULE C: REFERENCE MATERIALS

NFPA Guide on Hazardous Materials
CHRIS Condensed Guide to Chemical Hazards
Dangerous Properties of Industrial Materials (Sax)
NIOSH pocket Guide to Chemical Hazards
TLVs for Chemical Substances & Physical Agents in the Work
Environment

SCHEDULE D: FIELD SUPPORT KIT

Binoculars (2, 7 x 35mm wide angle)	Rangefinder (2)
Spotting scope	Stereoscopes
Compass (2)	Hand level (2)
Hand calculator (2)	Cassette recorder

SCHEDULE E: SOIL SAMPLING SET

Soil auger
Power head (electric)
Replacement tips for tube samplers
Scoops for bottom sediments
Stainless steel pipe section
Electrical resistivity apparatus
Post hole digger
Shovel

Auger extensions
Soil sample tubes
Wet, heavy duty tips
Labels
Logbooks for soil profiles
Stainless steel spoons
Pick-ax
Stainless steel pans

SCHEDULE F: WATER SAMPLEING SET

Weighted bottle sampler
Glass & polyethylene containers
Suction devices (hand pumps)
Cased thermometers/thermistors
Dissolved oxygen meter

Pond sampler
Scoops and dippers
Water level indicator
Teflon bailer
Conductivity meter

SCHEDULE G: AIR SAMPLING SET

Colorimetric indicator tubes
Impinger tubes
Particulate samplers
Wind speed indicator
Barometric pressure indicator

Hi-Vol sampler
Carbon adsorption tubes
Wind direction indicator
Temperature indicator
Temperature indicator

Chapter 9—CHEMICAL PROTECTIVE CLOTHING

I.   INTRODUCTION

A. The purpose of chemical protective clothing and equipment is to shield or isolate individuals from the chemical, physical, and biological

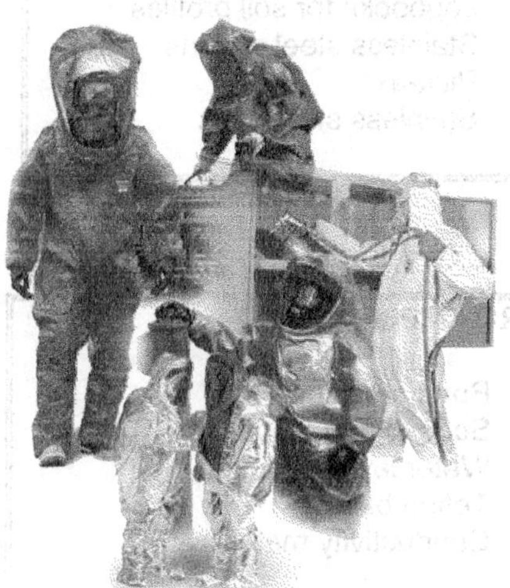

hazards that may be encountered during hazardous materials operations. During chemical operations, it is not always apparent when exposure occurs. Many chemicals pose invisible hazards and offer no warning properties.

B. These guidelines describe the various types of clothing that are appropriate for use in various chemical operations, and provides recommendations in their selection and use. The final paragraph discusses heat stress and other key physiological factors that must be considered in connection with protective clothing use.

C. It is important that protective clothing users realize that no single combination of protective equipment and clothing is capable of protecting you against all hazards. Thus protective clothing should be used in conjunction with other protective methods. For example, engineering or administrative controls to limit chemical contact with personnel should always be considered as an alternative measure for preventing chemical exposure. The use of protective clothing can itself create significant wearer hazards, such as heat stress, physical and psychological stress, in addition to impaired vision, mobility, and communication. In general, the greater the level of chemical protective clothing, the greater the associated risks. For any given situation, equipment and clothing should be selected that provide an adequate level of protection. Overprotection as well as under-protection can be hazardous and should be avoided.

II.   DESCRIPTIONS

PROTECTIVE CLOTHING APPLICATIONS.

Protective clothing must be worn whenever the wearer faces potential hazards arising from chemical exposure. Some examples include:

- Emergency response;
- Chemical manufacturing and process industries;
- Hazardous waste site cleanup and disposal;
- Asbestos removal and other particulate operations; and
- Agricultural application of pesticides.

Within each application, there are several operations which require chemical protective clothing. For example, in emergency response, the following activities dictate chemical protective clothing use:

- **Site Survey:** The initial investigation of a hazardous materials incident; these situations are usually characterized by a large degree of uncertainty and mandate the highest levels of protection.
- **Rescue:** Entering a hazardous materials area for the purpose of removing an exposure victim; special considerations must be given to how the selected protective clothing may affect the ability of the wearer to carry out rescue and to the contamination of the victim.
- **Spill Mitigation:** Entering a hazardous materials area to prevent a potential spill or to reduce the hazards from an existing spill (i.e., applying a chlorine kit on railroad tank car). Protective clothing must accommodate the required tasks without sacrificing adequate protection.
- **Emergency Monitoring:** Outfitting personnel in protective clothing for the primary purpose of observing a hazardous materials incident without entry into the spill site. This may be applied to monitoring contract activity for spill cleanup.
- **Decontamination:** Applying decontamination procedures to personnel or equipment leaving the site; in general a lower level of protective clothing is used by personnel involved in decontamination.

THE CLOTHING ENSEMBLE. The approach in selecting personal protective clothing must encompass an "ensemble" of clothing and equipment items which are easily integrated to provide both an appropriate level of protection and still allow one to carry out activities involving chemicals. In many cases, simple protective clothing by itself may be sufficient to prevent chemical exposure, such as wearing gloves in combination with a splash apron and faceshield (or safety goggles).

The following is a checklist of components that may form the chemical protective ensemble:

- Protective clothing (suit, coveralls, hoods, gloves, boots);
- Respiratory equipment (SCBA, combination SCBA/SAR, air purifying respirators);
- Cooling system (ice vest, air circulation, water circulation);
- Communications device;
- Head protection;
- Eye protection;
- Ear protection;
- Inner garment; and
- Outer protection (overgloves, overboots, flashcover).

Factors that affect the selection of ensemble components include:

- How each item accommodates the integration of other ensemble components. Some ensemble components may be incompatible due to how they are worn (e.g., some SCBA's may not fit within a particular chemical protective suit or allow acceptable mobility when worn).
- The ease of interfacing ensemble components without sacrificing required performance (e.g. a poorly fitting overglove that greatly reduces wearer dexterity).
- Limiting the number of equipment items to reduce donning time and complexity (e.g. some communications devices are built into SCBA's which as a unit are NIOSH certified).

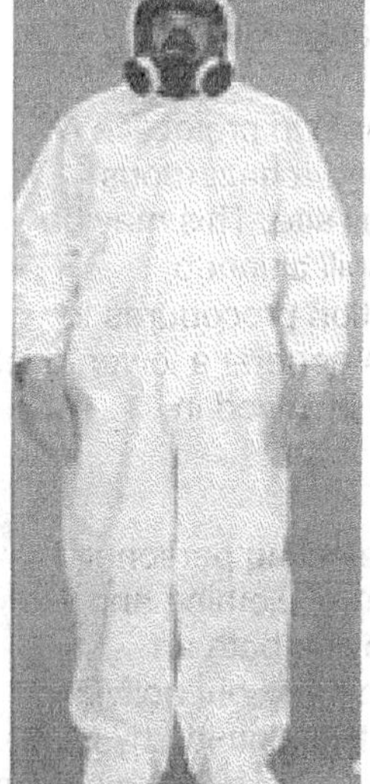

LEVEL OF PROTECTION.

Table VIII: 1-1 lists ensemble components based on the widely used *EPA Levels of Protection: Levels A, B, C, and D.* These lists can be used as the starting point for ensemble creation; however, each ensemble must be tailored to the specific situation in order to provide the most appropriate level of protection. For example, if an emergency response activity involves a highly contaminated area or if the potential of contamination is high, it may be advisable to wear a disposable covering such as Tyvek coveralls or PVC splash suits, over the protective ensemble.

TABLE VIII: 1-1. EPA LEVELS OF PROTECTION

LEVEL A:

Vapor protective suit (meets NFPA 1991)
Pressure-demand, full-face SCBA
Inner chemical-resistant gloves, chemical-resistant safety boots, two-way radio communication

OPTIONAL: Cooling system, outer gloves, hard hat

Protection Provided: Highest available level of respiratory, skin, and eye protection from solid, liquid and gaseous chemicals.

Used When: The chemical(s) have been identified and have high level of hazards to respiratory system, skin and eyes. Substances are present with known or suspected skin toxicity or carcinogenity. Operations must be conducted in confined or poorly ventilated areas.

Limitations: Protective clothing must resist permeation by the chemical or mixtures present. Ensemble items must allow integration without loss of performance.

LEVEL B:

Liquid splash-protective suit (meets NFPA 1992)
Pressure-demand, full-facepiece SCBA
Inner chemical-resistant gloves, chemical-resistant safety boots, two-way radio communications
Hard hat.

OPTIONAL: Cooling system, outer gloves

Protection Provided: Provides same level of respiratory protection as Level A, but less skin protection. Liquid splash protection, but no protection against chemical vapors or gases.

Used When: The chemical(s) have been identified but do not require a high level of skin protection. Initial site surveys are required until higher levels of hazards are identified. The primary hazards associated with site entry are from liquid and not vapor contact.

Limitations: Protective clothing items must resist penetration by the chemicals or mixtures present. Ensemble items must allow integration without loss of performance.

LEVEL C:

Support Function Protective Garment (meets NFPA 1993)
Full-facepiece, air-purifying, canister-equipped respirator
Chemical resistant gloves and safety boots
Two-way communications system, hard hat
OPTIONAL: Faceshield, escape SCBA

Protection Provided: The same level of skin protection as Level B, but a lower level of respiratory protection. Liquid splash protection but no protection to chemical vapors or gases.

Used When: Contact with site chemical(s) will not affect the skin. Air contaminants have been identified and concentrations measured. A canister is available which can remove the contaminant. The site and its hazards have been completely characterized.

Limitations: Protective clothing items must resist penetration by the chemical or mixtures present. Chemical airborne concentration must be less than IDLH levels. The atmosphere must contain at Least 19.5% oxygen.

Not Acceptable for Chemical Emergency Response

LEVEL D:

Coveralls, safety boots/shoes, safety glasses or chemical splash goggles

OPTIONAL: Gloves, escape SCBA, face-shield

Protection Provided: No respiratory protection, minimal skin protection.

Used When: The atmosphere contains no known hazard. Work functions preclude splashes, immersion, potential for inhalation, or direct contact with hazard chemicals.

Limitations: This level should not be worn in the Hot Zone. The atmosphere must contain at least 19.5% oxygen.

Not Acceptable for Chemical Emergency Response

The type of equipment used and the overall level of protection should be reevaluated periodically as the amount of information about the chemical situation or process increases, and when workers are required to perform different tasks. Personnel should upgrade or downgrade their level of protection only with concurrence with the site supervisor, safety officer, or plant industrial hygienist.

The recommendations in Table VIII:1-1 serve only as guidelines. It is important for you to realize that selecting items by how they are designed or configured alone is not sufficient to ensure adequate protection. In other words, just having the right components to form an ensemble is not enough. The EPA levels of protection do not define what performance the selected clothing or equipment must offer. Many of these considerations are described in the "limiting criteria" column of Table VIII: 1-1. Additional factors relevant to the various clothing and equipment items are described in subsequent Paragraphs.

ENSEMBLE SELECTION FACTORS.

Chemical Hazards. Chemicals present a variety of hazards such as toxicity, corrosiveness, flammability, reactivity, and oxygen deficiency. Depending on the chemicals present, any combination of hazards may exist.

Physical Environment. Chemical exposure can happen anywhere: in industrial settings, on the highways, or in residential areas. It may occur either indoors or outdoors; the environment may be extremely hot, cold, or moderate; the exposure site may be relatively uncluttered or rugged, presenting a number of physical hazards; chemical handling activities may involve entering confined spaces, heavy lifting, climbing a ladder, or crawling on the ground. The choice of ensemble components must account for these conditions.

Duration of Exposure. The protective qualities of ensemble components may be limited to certain exposure levels (e.g. material chemical resistance, air supply). The decision for ensemble use time must be made assuming the worst case exposure so that safety margins can be applied to increase the protection available to the worker.

Protective Clothing or Equipment Available. Hopefully, an array of different clothing or equipment is available to workers to meet all intended applications. Reliance on one particular clothing or equipment item may severely limit a facility's ability to handle a broad range of chemical exposures. In its acquisition of equipment and clothing, the safety department or other responsible authority should attempt to provide a high degree of flexibility while choosing protective clothing and equipment that is easily integrated and provides protection against each conceivable hazard.

CLASSIFICATION OF PROTECTIVE CLOTHING.

Personal protective clothing includes the following:

- Fully encapsulating suits;
- Nonencapsulating suits;
- Gloves, boots, and hoods;
- Firefighter's protective clothing;
- Proximity, or approach clothing;
- Blast or fragmentation suits; and
- Radiation-protective suits.

Firefighter turnout clothing, proximity gear, blast suits, and radiation suits by themselves are not acceptable for providing adequate protection from hazardous chemicals.

Table VIII:1-2 describes various types of protection clothing available, details the type of protection they offer, and lists factors to consider in their selection and use.

TABLE VIII: 1-2. TYPES OF PROTECTIVE CLOTHING FOR FULL BODY PROTECTION

Description	Type of Protection	Use Considerations
Fully encapsulating suit One-piece garment. Boots and gloves may be integral, attached and replaceable, or separate.	Protects against splashes, dust gases, and vapors.	Does not allow body heat to escape. May contribute to heat stress in wearer, particularly if worn in conjunction with a closed-circuit SCBA; a cooling garment may be needed. Impairs worker mobility, vision, and communication.
Nonencapsulating suit Jacket, hood, pants or bib overalls, and one-piece coveralls.	Protects against splashes, dust, and other materials but not against gases and vapors. Does not protect parts of head or neck.	Do not use where gas-tight or pervasive splashing protection is required. May contribute to heat stress in wearer. Tape-seal connections between pant cuffs and boots and between gloves and sleeves.
Aprons, leggings, and sleeve protectors Fully sleeved and gloved apron. Separate coverings for arms and legs. Commonly worn over nonencapsulating suit.	Provides additional splash protection of chest, forearms, and legs.	Whenever possible, should be used over a nonencapsulating suit to minimize potential heat stress. Useful for sampling, labeling, and analysis operations. Should be used only when there is a low probability of total body contact with contaminants.
Firefighters' protective clothing Gloves, helmet, running or bunker coat, running or bunker pants (NFPA No. 1971, 1972, 1973, and boots (1974).	Protects against heat, hot water, and some particles. Does not protect against gases and vapors, or chemical permeation or degradation. NFPA Standard No. 1971 specifies that a garment consists of an outer shell, an inner liner and a vapor barrier with a minimum water penetration of 25 lb/in^2 (1.8 kg/cm^2) to prevent passage of hot	Decontamination is difficult. Should not be worn in areas where protection against gases, vapors, chemical splashes or permeation is required.

water.

Proximity garment (approach suit) One- or two-piece overgarment with boot covers, gloves, and hood of aluminized nylon or cotton fabric. Normally worn over other protective clothing, firefighters' bunker gear, or flame-retardant coveralls.	Protects against splashes, dust, gases, and vapors.	Does not allow body heat to escape. May contribute to heat stress in wearer, particularly if worn in conjunction with a closed-circuit SCBA; a cooling garment may be needed. Impairs worker mobility, vision, and communication.
Blast and fragmentation suit Blast and fragmentation vests and clothing, bomb blankets, and bomb carriers.	Provides some protection against very small detonations. Bomb blankets and baskets can help redirect a blast.	Does not provide for hearing protection.
Radiation-contamination protective suit Various types of protective clothing designed to prevent contamination of the body by radioactive particles.	Protects against alpha and beta particles. Does *not* protect against gamma radiation.	Designed to prevent skin contamination. If radiation is detected on site, consult an experienced radiation expert and evacuate personnel until the radiation hazard has been evaluated.
Flame/fire retardant coveralls Normally worn as an undergarment.	Provides protection from flash fires.	Adds bulk and may exacerbate heat stress problems and impair mobility

CLASSIFICATION OF CHEMICAL PROTECTIVE CLOTHING. Table VIII: 1-3 provides a listing of clothing classifications. Clothing can be classified by design, performance, and service life.

TABLE VIII: 1-3. CLASSIFICATION OF CHEMICAL PROTECTIVE CLOTHING

By Design	By Performance	By Service Life
gloves	particulate protection	single use
boots	liquid-splash protection	limited use
aprons, jackets, coveralls, full body suits	vapor protection	reusable

Design. Categorizing clothing by design is mainly a means for describing what areas of the body the clothing item is intended to protect.

In emergency response, hazardous waste site cleanup, and dangerous chemical operations, the only acceptable types of protective clothing include fully or totally encapsulating suits and nonencapsulating or "splash" suits plus accessory clothing items such as chemically resistant gloves or boots. These descriptions apply to how the clothing is designed and not to its performance.

Performance. The National Fire Protection Association (NFPA) has classified suits by their performance as:

<u>Vapor-protective suits</u> (NFPA Standard 1991) provide "gas-tight" integrity and are intended for response situations where no chemical contact is permissible. This type of suit would be equivalent to the clothing required in EPA's Level A.

<u>Liquid splash-protective suits</u> (NFPA Standard 1992) offer protection against liquid chemicals in the form of splashes, but not against continuous liquid contact or chemical vapors or gases. Essentially, the type of clothing would meet the EPA Level B needs. It is important to note, however, that by wearing liquid splash-protective clothing, the wearer accepts exposure to chemical vapors or gases because this clothing does not offer gas-tight performance. The use of duct tape to seal clothing interfaces does not provide the type of wearer encapsulation necessary for protection against vapors or gases.

<u>Support function protective garments</u> (NFPA Standard 1993) must also provide liquid splash protection but offer limited physical protection. These garments may comprise several separate protective clothing components (i.e., coveralls, hoods, gloves, and boots). They are intended for use in nonemergency, nonflammable situations where the chemical hazards have been completely characterized. Examples of support functions include proximity to chemical processes, decontamination, hazardous waste clean-up, and training. Support function protective garments should not be used in chemical emergency response or in situations where chemical hazards remain uncharacterized.

These <u>NFPA standards</u> define minimum performance requirements for the manufacture of chemical protective suits. Each standard requires rigorous testing of the suit and the materials that comprise the suit in terms of overall protection, chemical resistance, and physical properties.

Suits that are found compliant by an independent certification and testing organization may be labeled by the manufacturer as meeting the requirements of the respective NFPA standard. Manufacturers also have to supply documentation showing all test results and characteristics of their protective suits.

Protective clothing should completely cover both the wearer and his or her breathing apparatus. In general, respiratory protective equipment is not designed to resist chemical contamination. Level A protection (vapor-protective suits) require this configuration. Level B ensembles may be configured either with the SCBA on the outside or inside. However, it is strongly recommended that the wearer's respiratory equipment be worn inside the ensemble to prevent its failure and to reduce decontamination problems. Level C ensembles use cartridge or canister type respirators which are generally worn outside the clothing.

Service Life.

Clothing item service life is an end user decision depending on the costs and risks associated with clothing decontamination and reuse. For example, a Saranex/Tyvek garment may be designed to be a coverall (covering the wearer's torso, arms, and legs) intended for liquid splash protection, which is disposable after a single use.

Protective clothing may be labeled as:

- Reusable, for multiple wearings; or
- Disposable, for one-time use.

The distinctions between these types of clothing are both vague and complicated. Disposable clothing is generally lightweight and inexpensive. Reusable clothing is often more rugged and costly. Nevertheless, extensive contamination of any garment may render it disposable. The basis of this classification really depends on the costs involved in purchasing, maintaining, and reusing protective clothing versus the al ternative of disposal following exposure. If an end user can anticipate obtaining several uses out of a garment while still maintaining adequate protection from that garment at lower cost than its disposal, the suit becomes reusable. Yet, the key assumption in this determination is the viability of the garment following exposure. This issue is further discussed in the Paragraph on decontamination.

III.   PROTECTIVE CLOTHING SELECTION FACTORS.

CLOTHING DESIGN. Manufacturers sell clothing in a variety of styles and configurations.

Design Considerations.

- Clothing configuration;
- Components and options;
- Sizes;
- Ease of donning and doffing;
- Clothing construction;
- Accommodation of other selected ensemble equipment;
- Comfort; and
- Restriction of mobility.

MATERIAL CHEMICAL RESISTANCE. Ideally, the chosen material(s) must resist permeation, degradation, and penetration by the respective chemicals.

Permeation is the process by which a chemical dissolves in or moves through a material on a molecular basis. In most cases, there will be no visible evidence of chemicals permeating a material.

Permeation breakthrough time is the most common result used to assess material chemical compatibility. The rate of permeation is a function of several factors such as chemical concentration, material thickness, humidity, temperature, and pressure. Most material testing is done with 100% chemical over an extended exposure period. The time it takes chemical to permeate through the material is the breakthrough time. An acceptable material is one where the breakthrough time exceeds the expected period of garment use. However, temperature and pressure effects may enhance permeation and reduce the magnitude of this safety factor. For example, small increases in ambient temperature can significantly reduce breakthrough time and the protective barrier properties of a protective clothing material.

Degradation involves physical changes in a material as the result of a chemical exposure, use, or ambient conditions (e.g. sunlight). The most common observations of material degradation are discoloration, swelling, loss of physical strength, or deterioration.

Penetration is the movement of chemicals through zippers, seams, or imperfections in a protective clothing material.

It is important to note that no material protects against all chemicals and combinations of chemicals, and that no currently available material is an effective barrier to any prolonged chemical exposure.

Sources of information include:

- *Guidelines for the Selection of Chemical Protective Clothing,* 3rd Edition. This reference provides a matrix of clothing material recommendations for approximately 500 chemicals based on an evaluation of chemical resistance test data, vendor literature, and raw material suppliers. The major limitation for these guidelines are their presentation of recommendations by generic material class. Numerous test results have shown that similar materials from different manufacturers may give widely different performance. That is to say manufacturer A's butyl rubber glove may protect against chemical X, but a butyl glove made by manufacturer B may not.

- *Quick Selection Guide to Chemical Protective Clothing.* Pocket size guide that provides chemical resistance data and recommendations for 11 generic materials against over 400 chemicals. The guide is color-coded by material-chemical recommendation. As with the "Guidelines..." above, the major limitation of this reference is its dependence on generic data.

- Vendor data or recommendations. The best source of current information on material compatibility should be available from the manufacturer of the selected clothing. Many vendors supply charts which show actual test data or their own recommendations for specific chemicals. However, *unless vendor data or the recommendations are well documented, end users must approach this information with caution.* Material recommendations must be based on data obtained from tests performed to standard ASTM methods. Simple ratings of "poor," "good," or "excellent" give no indication of how the material may perform against various chemicals.

- Mixtures of chemicals can be significantly more aggressive towards protective clothing materials than any single chemical alone. One permeating chemical may pull another with it through the material. Very little data is available for chemical mixtures. Other situations may involve unidentified substances. In both the case of mixtures and unknowns, serious consideration must be given to deciding which protective clothing is selected. If clothing must be used without test data, garments with materials having the broadest chemical resistance should be worn, i.e. materials

which demonstrate the best chemical resistance against the
widest range of chemicals.

PHYSICAL PROPERTIES.

As with chemical resistance, manufacturer materials offer wide ranges of
physical qualities in terms of strength, resistance to physical hazards,
and operation in extreme environmental conditions. Comprehensive
manufacturing standards such as the NFPA Standards set specific limits
on these material properties, but only for limited applications, i.e.
emergency response.

End users in other applications may assess material physical properties
by posing the following questions:

- Does the material have sufficient strength to withstand the
  physical strength of the tasks at hand?
- Will the material resist tears, punctures, cuts, and abrasions?
- Will the material withstand repeated use after contamination and
  decontamination?
- Is the material flexible or pliable enough to allow end users to
  perform needed tasks?
- Will the material maintain its protective integrity and flexibility
  under hot and cold extremes?
- Is the material flame-resistant or self-extinguishing (if these
  hazards are present)?
- Are garment seams in the clothing constructed so they provide
  the same physical integrity as the garment material?

EASE OF DECONTAMINATION. The degree of difficulty in
decontaminating protective clothing may dictate whether disposable or
reusable clothing is used, or a combination of both.

COST. Protective clothing end users must endeavor to obtain the
broadest protective equipment they can buy with available resources to
meet their specific application.

CHEMICAL PROTECTIVE CLOTHING STANDARDS. Protective
clothing buyers may wish to specify clothing that meets specific
standards, such as 1910.120 or the NFPA standards (see Paragraph on
classification by performance). The NFPA Standards do not apply to all
forms of protective clothing and applications.

## IV.	GENERAL GUIDELINES.

DECIDE IF THE CLOTHING ITEM IS INTENDED TO PROVIDE VAPOR, LIQUID-SPLASH, OR PARTICULATE PROTECTION.

<u>Vapor protective suits</u> also provide liquid splash and particulate protection. Liquid splash protective garments also provide particulate protection. Many garments may be labeled as totally encapsulating but do not provide gas-tight integrity due to inadequate seams or closures. Gas-tight integrity can only be determined by performing a pressure or inflation test and a leak detection test of the respective protective suit. This test involves:

- Closing off suit exhalation valves;
- Inflating the suit to a prespecified pressure; and
- Observing whether the suit holds the above pressure for a designated period.

ASTM Standard Practice F1052 (1987 Edition) offers a procedure for conducting this test.

<u>Splash suits</u> must still cover the entire body when combined with the respirator, gloves, and boots. Applying duct tape to a splash suit does not make it protect against vapors. Particulate protective suits may not need to cover the entire body, depending on the hazards posed by the particulate. In general, gloves, boots and some form of face protection are required. Clothing items may only be needed to cover a limited area of the body such as gloves on hands. The nature of the hazards and the expected exposure will determine if clothing should provide partial or full body protection.

DETERMINE IF THE CLOTHING ITEM PROVIDES FULL BODY PROTECTION.

<u>Vapor-protective or totally encapsulating suit</u> will meet this requirement by passing gas-tight integrity tests.

- Liquid splash-protective suits are generally sold incomplete (i.e. fewer gloves and boots).
- Missing clothing items must be obtained separately and match or exceed the performance of the garment.
- Buying a PVC glove for a PVC splash suit does not mean that you obtain the same level of protection. This determination must be made by comparing chemical resistance data.

EVALUATE MANUFACTURER CHEMICAL RESISTANCE DATA PROVIDED WITH THE CLOTHING.

1. Manufacturers of vapor-protective suits should provide permeation resistance data for their products, while liquid and particulate penetration resistance data should accompany liquid splash and particulate protective garments respectively. Ideally data should be provided for every primary material in the suit or clothing item. For suits, this includes the garment, visor, gloves, boots, and seams.

2. Permeation data should include the following:

   - Chemical name;
   - Breakthrough time (shows how soon the chemical permeates);
   - Permeation rate (shows the rate that the chemical comes through);
   - System sensitivity (allows comparison of test results from different laboratories); and
   - A citation that the data was obtained in accordance with ASTM Standard Test Method F739-85.

3. If no data are provided or if the data lack any one of the above items, the manufacturer should be asked to supply the missing data. Manufacturers that provide only numerical or qualitative ratings must support their recommendations with complete test data.

4. Liquid penetration data should include a pass or fail determination for each chemical listed, and a citation that testing was conducted in accordance with ASTM Standard Test Method F903-86. Protective suits which are certified to NFPA 1991 or NFPA 1992 will meet all of the above requirements.

5. Particulate penetration data should show some measure of material efficiency in preventing particulate penetration in terms of particulate type or size and percentage held out. Unfortunately, no standard tests are available in this area and end users may have little basis for company products.

6. Suit materials which show no breakthrough or no penetration to a large number of chemicals are likely to have a broad range of chemical resistance. (Breakthrough times greater than one hour are usually considered to be an indication of acceptable performance.) Manufacturers should provide data on the ASTM

Standard Guide F1001-86 chemicals. These 15 liquid and 6
gaseous chemicals listed in Table VIII:1-4 below represent a
cross-section of different chemical classes and challenges for
protective clothing materials. Manufacturers should also provide
test data on other chemicals as well. If there are specific
chemicals within your operating area that have not been tested,
ask the manufacturer for test data on these chemicals.

Chemical	Class
Acetone	Ketone
Acetonitrile	Nitrile
Ammonia	Strong base (gas)
1,3-Butadiene	Olefin (gas)
Carbpm Dosi;fode	Sulfur-containing organic
Chlorine	Inorganic gas
Dichloromethane	Chlorinated hydrocarbon
Diethylamine	Amine
Dimethyl formamide	Amide
Ethyl Acetate	Ester
Ethyl Oxide	Oxygen heterocyclic gas
Hexane	Aliphatic hydrocarbon
Hydrogen Chloride	Acid gas
Methanol	Alcohol
Methyl Chloride	Chlorinated hydrocarbon (gas)
Nitrobenzene	Nitrogen-containing organic
Sodium Hydroxide	Inorganic base
Sulfuric Acid	Inorganic acid
Tetrachloroethylene	Chlorinated hydrocarbon
Tetrahydrofuran	Oxygen heterocyclic
Toluene	Aromatic hydrocarbon

OBTAIN AND EXAMINE THE MANUFACTURER'S INSTRUCTION OR TECHNICAL MANUAL.

This manual should document all the features of the clothing, particularly suits, and describe what material(s) are used in its construction. It should cite specific limitations for the clothing and what restrictions apply to its use. Procedures and recommendations should be supplied for at least the following:

- Donning and doffing;
- Inspection, maintenance, and storage;
- Decontamination; and
- Use.

The manufacturer's instructions should be thorough enough to allow the end users to wear and use the clothing without a large number of questions.

OBTAIN AND INSPECT SAMPLE CLOTHING ITEM GARMENTS.
Examine the quality of clothing construction and other features that will
impact its wearing. The questions listed under "Protective Clothing
Selection Factors, Clothing Design" should be considered. If possible,
representative clothing items should be obtained in advance and
inspected prior to purchase, and discussed with someone who has
experience in their use. It is also helpful to try out representative
garments prior to purchase by suiting personnel in the garment and
having them run through exercises to simulate expected activities.

FIELD SELECTION OF CHEMICAL PROTECTIVE CLOTHING.

Even when end users have gone through a very careful selection
process, a number of situations will arise when no information is
available to judge whether their protective clothing will provide adequate
protection. These situations include:

- Chemicals that have not been tested with the garment materials;
- Mixtures of two or more different chemicals;
- Chemicals that cannot be readily identified;
- Extreme environmental conditions (hot temperatures); and
- Lack of data in all clothing components (e.g. seams, visors).

Testing material specimens using newly developed field test kits may
offer one means for making an on-site clothing selection. A portable test
kit has been developed by the EPA using a simple weight loss method
that allows field qualification of protective clothing materials within one
hour. Use of this kit may overcome the absence of data and provide
additional criteria for clothing selection.

*Selection of chemical protective clothing is a complex task and should be
performed by personnel with both extensive training and experience.*

Under all conditions, clothing should be selected by evaluating its
performance characteristics against the requirements and limitations
imposed by the application.

V.   MANAGEMENT PROGRAM.

WRITTEN MANAGEMENT PROGRAM.

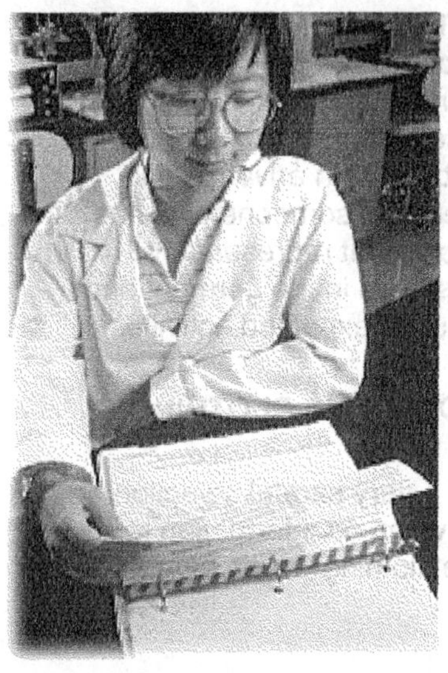

A written Chemical Protective Clothing Management Program should be established by all end users who routinely select and use protective clothing. Reference should be made to 1910.120 for those covered.

The written management program should include policy statements, procedures, and guidelines. Copies should be made available to all personnel who may use protective clothing in the course of their duties or job. Technical data on clothing, maintenance manuals, relevant regulations, and other essential information should also be made available.

The two basic objectives of any management program should be to protect the wearer from safety and health hazards, and to prevent injury to the wearer from incorrect use and/or malfunction of the chemical protective clothing. To accomplish these goals, a comprehensive management program should include: hazard identification; medical monitoring; environmental surveillance; selection, use, maintenance, and decontamination of chemical protective clothing; and training.

PROGRAM REVIEW AND EVALUATION. The management program should be reviewed at least annually. Elements which should be considered in the review include:

- The number of person-hours that personnel wear various forms of chemical protective clothing and other equipment;
- Accident and illness experience;
- Levels of exposure;
- Adequacy of equipment selection;
- Adequacy of the operational guidelines;
- Adequacy of decontamination, cleaning, inspection, maintenance, and storage programs;
- Adequacy and effectiveness of training and fitting programs;
- Coordination with overall safety and health program;
- The degree of fulfillment of program objectives;
- The adequacy of program records;
- Recommendations for program improvement and modification; and

- Program costs.

The results of the program evaluation should be made available to all end users and presented to top management so that program changes may be implemented.

TYPES OF STANDARD OPERATING PROCEDURES. Personal protective clothing and equipment can offer a high degree of protection only if it is used properly. Standard Operating Procedures (SOP's) should be established for all workers involved in handling hazardous chemicals. Areas that should be addressed include:

- Selection of protective ensemble components;
- Protective clothing and equipment donning, doffing, and use;
- Decontamination procedures;
- Inspection, storage, and maintenance of protective clothing/equipment; and
- Training.

SELECTION OF PROTECTIVE CLOTHING COMPONENTS.

Protective clothing and equipment SOP's must take into consideration the factors presented in the Clothing Ensemble and Protective Clothing Applications Paragraphs of this chapter. All clothing and equipment selections should provide a decision tree that relates chemical hazards and information to levels of protection and performance needed.

Responsibility in selecting appropriate protective clothing should be vested in a specific individual who is trained in both chemical hazards and protective clothing use such as a safety officer or industrial hygienist. Only chemical protective suits labeled as compliant with the appropriate performance requirements should be used. In cases where the chemical hazards are known in advance or encountered routinely, clothing selection should be predetermined. That is, specific clothing items should be identified in specific chemical operations without the opportunity for individual selection of other clothing items.

VI. CLOTHING DONNING, DOFFING, AND USE.

The procedures below are given for vapor protective or liquid-splash
protective suit ensembles and should be included in the training
program.

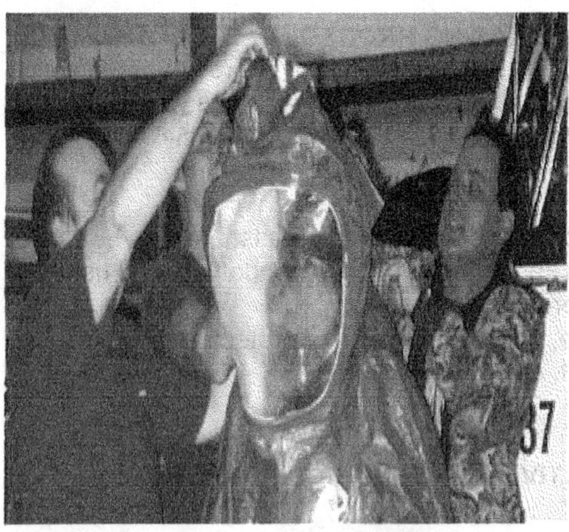

**DONNING THE
ENSEMBLE.**

A routine should be
established and
practiced periodically for
donning the various
ensemble
configurations that a
facility or team may use.
Assistance should be
provided for donning
and doffing since these
operations are difficult
to perform alone, and
solo efforts may
increase the possibility of ensemble damage.

Table VIII:1-5 below lists sample procedures for donning a totally
encapsulating suit/SCBA ensemble. These procedures should be
modified depending on the suit and accessory equipment used. The
procedures assume the wearer has previous training in respirator use
and decontamination procedures.

Once the equipment has been donned, its fit should be evaluated. If the
clothing is too small, it will restrict movement, increase the likelihood of
tearing the suit material, and accelerate wearer fatigue. If the clothing is
too large, the possibility of snagging the material is increased, and the
dexterity and coordination of the wearer may be compromised. In either
case, the wearer should be recalled and better-fitting clothing provided.

<h1 style="text-align:center">TABLE VIII: 1-5. SAMPLE DONNING PROCEDURES</h1>

1.   Inspect clothing and respiratory equipment before donning (see Paragraph on Inspection).

2.   Adjust hard hat or headpiece if worn, to fit user's head.

3.   Open back closure used to change air tank (if suit has one) before donning suit.

4.   Standing or sitting, step into the legs of the suit; ensure proper placement of the feet within the suit; then gather the suit around the waist.

5.   Put on chemical-resistant safety boots over the feet of the suit. Tape the leg cuff over the tops of the boots. If additional chemical-resistant safety boots are required, put these on now.   Some one-piece suits have heavy-soled protective feet. With these suits, wear short, chemical resistant safety boots inside the suit.

6.   Put on air tank and harness assembly of the SCBA. Don the facepiece and adjust it to be secure, but comfortable. Do not connect the breathing hose. Open valve on air tank.

7.   Perform negative and positive respirator facepiece seal test procedures. To conduct a negative-pressure test, close the inlet part with the palm of the hand or squeeze the breathing tube so it does not pass air, and gently inhale for about 10 seconds. Any inward rushing of air indicates a poor fit. Note that a leaking facepiece may be drawn tightly to the face to form a good seal, giving a false indication of adequate fit.
To conduct a positive-pressure test, gently exhale while covering the exhalation valve to ensure that a positive pressure can be built up. Failure to build a positive pressure indicates a poor fit.

8.   Depending on type of suit: Put on long-sleeved inner gloves (similar to surgical gloves). Secure gloves to sleeves, for suits with detachable gloves (if not done prior to entering the suit).   Additional overgloves, worn over attached suit gloves, may be donned later.

9.   Put sleeves of suit over arms as assistant pulls suit up and over the SCBA. Have assistant adjust suit around SCBA and shoulders to ensure unrestricted motion.

10.   Put on hard hat, if needed.

11.   Raise hood over head carefully so as not to disrupt face seal of SCBA mask. Adjust hood to give satisfactory comfort.

12.   Begin to secure the suit by closing all fasteners on opening until there is only adequate room to connect the breathing hose. Secure all belts and/or adjustable leg, head, and waistbands.

13.   Connect the breathing hose while opening the main valve.

14.   Have assistant first ensure that wearer is breathing properly and then make final closure of the suit.

15.   Have assistant check all closures.

16.   Have assistant observe the wearer for a period of time to ensure that the wearer is comfortable, psychologically stable, and that the equipment is functioning properly.

17.   DOFFING AN ENSEMBLE.

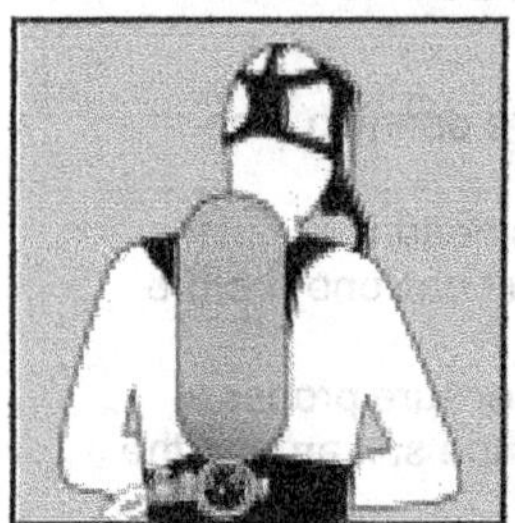

Exact procedures for removing a totally encapsulating suit/SCBA ensemble must be established and followed in order to prevent contaminant migration from the response scene and transfer of contaminants to the wearer's body, the doffing assistant, and others.

Sample doffing procedures are provided in Table VIII:1-6 below. These procedures should be performed only after decontamination of the suited end user. They require a suitably attired assistance. Throughout the procedures, both wearer and assistant should avoid any direct contact with the outside surface of the suit.

TABLE VIII: 1-6. SAMPLE DOFFING PROCEDURES

If sufficient air supply is available to allow appropriate decontamination before removal

1.   Remove any extraneous or disposable clothing, boot covers, outer gloves, and tape.
2.   Have assistant loosen and remove the wearer's safety shoes or boots.
3.   Have assistant open the suit completely and lift the hood over the head of the wearer and rest it on top of the SCBA tank.
4.   Remove arms, one at a time, from suit. Once arms are free, have assistant lift the suit up and away from the SCBA backpack--avoiding any contact between the outside surface of the suit and the wearer's body--and lay the suit out flat behind the wearer. Leave internal gloves on, if any.
5.   Sitting, if possible, remove both legs from the suit.
6.   Follow procedure for doffing SCBA.
7.   After suit is removed, remove internal gloves by rolling them off the hand, inside out.
8.   Remove internal clothing and thoroughly cleanse the body.

If the low-pressure warning alarm has sounded, signifying that approximately 5 minutes of air remain:

9.   Remove disposable clothing.
10. Quickly scrub and hose off, especially around the entrance/exit zipper.
11. Open the zipper enough to allow access to the regulator and breathing hose.
12. Immediately attach an appropriate canister to the breathing hose (the type and fittings should be predetermined). Although this provides some

protection against any contamination still present, it voids the certification of the unit.

13. Follow Steps 1 through 8 of the regular doffing procedure above. Take extra care to avoid contaminating the assistant and the wearer.

USER MONITORING AND TRAINING.

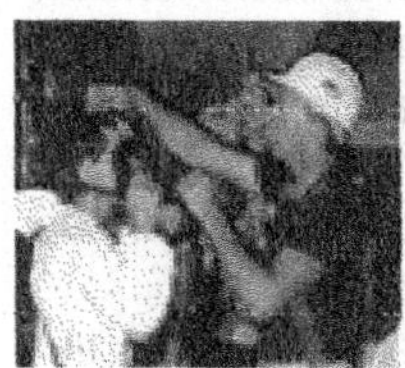
The wearer must understand all aspects of clothing/equipment operation and their limitations; this is especially important for fully encapsulating ensembles where misuse could potentially result in suffocation. During protective clothing use, end users should be encouraged to report any perceived problems or difficulties to their supervisor. These malfunctions include, but are not limited to:

- Degradation of the protection ensemble;
- Perception of odors;
- Skin irritation;
- Unusual residues on clothing material;
- Discomfort;
- Resistance to breathing;
- Fatigue due to respirator use;
- Interference with vision or communication;
- Restriction of movement; and
- Physiological responses such as rapid pulse, nausea, or chest pain.

Before end users undertake any activity in their chemical protective ensembles, the anticipated duration of use should be established. Several factors limit the length of a mission, including:

- Air supply consumption as affected by wearer work rate, fitness, body size, and breathing patterns;
- Suit ensemble permeation, degradation, and penetration by chemical contaminants, including expected leakage through suit or respirator exhaust valves (ensemble protection factor);
- Ambient temperature as it influences material chemical resistance and flexibility, suit and respirator exhaust valve performance, and wearer heat stress; and
- Coolant supply (if necessary).

VII. DECONTAMINATION PROCEDURES.

DEFINITION AND TYPES.

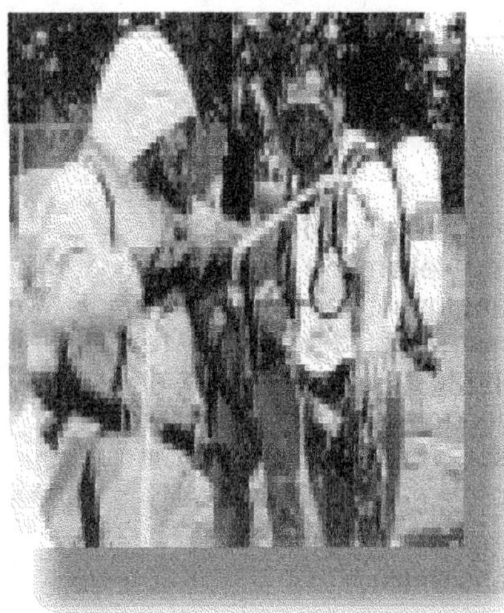

Decontamination is the process of removing or neutralizing contaminants that have accumulated on personnel and equipment. This process is critical to health and safety at hazardous material response sites. Decontamination protects end users from hazardous substances that may contaminate and eventually permeate the protective clothing, respiratory equipment, tools, vehicles, and other equipment used in the vicinity of the chemical hazard; it protects all plant or site personnel by minimizing the transfer of harmful materials into clean areas; it helps prevent mixing of incompatible chemicals; and it protects the community by preventing uncontrolled transportation of contaminants from the site.

There are two types of decontamination:

1. **Gross decontamination:** To allow end user to safely exit or doff the chemical protective clothing.
2. **Decontamination** for reuse of chemical protective clothing.

PREVENTION OF CONTAMINATION. The first step in decontamination is to establish Standard Operating Procedures that minimize contact with chemicals and thus the potential for contamination. For example:

- Stress work practices that minimize contact with hazardous substances (e.g. do not walk through areas of obvious contamination, do not directly touch potentially hazardous substances).
- Use remote sampling, handling, and container-opening techniques (e.g. drum grapples, pneumatic impact wrenches).
- Protect monitoring and sampling instruments by bagging. Make openings in the bags for sample ports and sensors that must contact site materials.

- Wear disposable outer garments and use disposable equipment where appropriate.
- Cover equipment and tools with a strippable coating that can be removed during decontamination.
- Encase the source of contaminants, e.g. with plastic sheeting or overpacks.
- Ensure all closures and ensemble component interfaces are completely secured; and that no open pockets that could serve to collect contaminant are present.

TYPES OF CONTAMINATION.

Surface Contaminants. Surface contaminants may be easy to detect and remove.

Permeated Contaminants. Contaminants that have permeated a material are difficult or impossible to detect and remove. If contaminants that have permeated a material are not removed by decontamination, they may continue to permeate the material where they can cause an unexpected exposure.

Four major factors affect the extent of permeation:

1. **Contact time.** The longer a contaminant is in contact with an object, the greater the probability and extent of permeation. For this reason, minimizing contact time is one of the most important objectives of a decontamination program.
2. **Concentration.** Molecules flow from areas of high concentration to areas of low concentration. As concentrations of chemicals increase, the potential for permeation of personal protective clothing increases.
3. **Temperature.** An increase in temperature generally increases the permeation rate of contaminants.
4. **Physical state of chemicals.** As a rule, gases, vapors, and low-viscosity liquids tend to permeate more readily than high-viscosity liquids or solids.

DECONTAMINATION METHODS.

Decontamination methods either (1) physically remove contaminants; (2) inactivate contaminants by chemical detoxification or disinfection/sterilization; or (3) remove contaminants by a combination of both physical and chemical means.

In general, gross decontamination is accomplished using detergents (surfactants) in water combined with a physical scrubbing action. This process will remove most forms of surface contamination including dusts, many inorganic chemicals, and some organic chemicals. Soapy water scrubbing of protective suits may not be effective in removing oily or tacky organic substances (e.g. PCB's in transformer oil). Furthermore, this form of decontamination is unlikely to remove any contamination that has permeated or penetrated the suit materials. Using organic solvents such as petroleum distillates may allow easier removal of heavy organic contamination but may result in other problems, including:

- Permeation into clothing components, pulling the contaminant with it;
- Spreading localized contaminant into other areas of the clothing; and
- Generating large volumes of contaminated solvents that require disposal.

One promising method for removing internal or matrix contamination is the forced circulation of heated air over clothing items for extended periods of time. This allows many organic chemicals to migrate out of the materials and evaporate into the heated air. The process does require, however, that the contaminating chemicals be volatile. Additionally, low level heat may accelerate the removal of plasticizer from garment materials and affect the adhesives involved in garment seams.

Unfortunately, both manufacturers and protective clothing authorities provide few specific recommendations for decontamination. There is no definitive list with specific methods recommended for specific chemicals and materials. Much depends on the individual chemical-material combination involved.

TESTING THE EFFECTIVENESS OF DECONTAMINATION.

Protective clothing or equipment reuse depends on demonstrating that adequate decontamination has taken place. Decontamination methods vary in their effectiveness and unfortunately there are no completely accurate methods for nondestructively evaluating clothing or equipment contamination levels.

Methods which may assist in a determination include:

- Visual examination of protective clothing for signs of discoloration, corrosive effects, or any degradation of external

materials. However, many contaminants do not leave any visible
evidence.

- Wipe sampling of external surfaces for subsequent analysis; this
  may or may not be effective for determining levels of surface
  contamination and depends heavily on the material-chemical
  combination. These methods will not detect permeated
  contamination.

- Evaluation of the cleaning solution. This method cannot quantify
  clean method effectiveness since the original contamination
  levels are unknown. The method can only show if chemical has
  been removed by the cleaning solution. If a number of garments
  have been contaminated, it may be advisable to sacrifice one
  garment for destructive testing by a qualified laboratory with
  analysis of contamination levels on and inside the garment.

DECONTAMINATION PLAN.

A decontamination plan should be developed and set up before any
personnel or equipment are allowed to enter areas where the potential
for exposure to hazardous substances exists. The decontamination plan
should:

- Determine the number and layout of decontamination stations;

- Determine the decontamination equipment needed;

- Determine appropriate decontamination methods;

- Establish procedures to prevent contamination of clean areas;

- Establish methods and procedures to minimize wearer contact
  with contaminants during removal of personal protective clothing;
  and

- Establish methods for disposing of clothing and equipment that
  are not completely decontaminated.

The plan should be revised whenever the type of personal protective
clothing or equipment changes, the use conditions change, or the
chemical hazards are reassessed based on new information.

The decontamination process should consist of a series of procedures
performed in a specific sequence. For chemical protective ensembles,
outer, more heavily contaminated items (e.g. outer boots and gloves)
should be decontaminated and removed first, followed by

decontamination and removal of inner, less contaminated items (e.g. jackets and pants). Each procedure should be performed at a separate station in order to prevent cross contamination. The sequence of stations is called the decontamination line.

Stations should be separated physically to prevent cross contamination and should be arranged in order of decreasing contamination, preferably in a straight line. Separate flow patterns and stations should be provided to isolate workers from different contamination zones containing incompatible wastes. Entry and exit points to exposed areas should be conspicuously marked. Dressing stations for entry to the decontamination area should be separate from redressing areas for exit from the decontamination area. Personnel who wish to enter clean areas of the decontamination facility, such as locker rooms, should be completely decontaminated.

All equipment used for decontamination must be decontaminated and/or disposed of properly. Buckets, brushes, clothing, tools, and other contaminated equipment should be collected, placed in containers, and labeled. Also, all spent solutions and wash water should be collected and disposed of properly. Clothing that is not completely decontaminated should be placed in plastic bags, pending further decontamination and/or disposal.

Decontamination of workers who initially come in contact with personnel and equipment leaving exposure or contamination areas will require more protection from contaminants than decontamination workers who are assigned to the last station in the decontamination line. In some cases, decontamination personnel should wear the same levels of protective clothing as workers in the exposure or contaminated areas. In other cases, decontamination personnel may be sufficiently protected by wearing one level lower protection (e.g. wearing Level B protection while decontaminating workers who are wearing Level A).

DECONTAMINATION FOR PROTECTIVE CLOTHING REUSE. Due to the difficulty in assessing contamination levels in chemical protective clothing before and after exposure, the responsible supervisor or safety professional must determine if the respective clothing can be reused. This decision involves considerable risk in determining clothing to be contaminant-free. Reuse can be considered if, in the estimate of the supervisor:

- No "significant" exposures have occurred.

- Decontamination methods have been successful in reducing contamination levels to safe or acceptable concentrations.

Contamination by known or suspected carcinogens should warrant automatic disposal. Use of disposable suits is highly recommended when extensive contamination is expected.

EMERGENCY DECONTAMINATION.

In addition to routine decontamination procedures, emergency decontamination procedures must be established. In an emergency, the primary concern is to prevent the loss of life or severe injury to personnel. If immediate medical treatment is required to save a life, decontamination should be delayed until the victim is stabilized. If decontamination can be performed without interfering with essential life-saving techniques or first aid, or if a worker has been contaminated with an extremely toxic or corrosive material that could cause severe injury or loss of life, decontamination should be continued.

If an emergency due to a heat-related illness develops, protective clothing should be removed from the victim as soon as possible to reduce the heat stress. During an emergency, provisions must also be made for protecting medical personnel and disposing of contaminated clothing and equipment.

VIII. INSPECTION, STORAGE, AND MAINTENANCE.

The end user in donning protective clothing and equipment must take all necessary steps to ensure that the protective ensemble will perform as expected. During emergencies is not the right time to discover discrepancies in the protective clothing. Teach end user care for his clothing and other protective equipment in the same manner as parachutists care for parachutes. Following a standard program for inspection, proper storage, and maintenance along with realizing protective clothing/equipment limitations is the best way to avoid chemical exposure during emergency response.

INSPECTION.

An effective chemical protective clothing inspection program should feature five different inspections:

1. Inspection and operational testing of equipment received as new from the factory or distributor.
2. Inspection of equipment as it is selected for a particular chemical operation.
3. Inspection of equipment after use or training and prior to maintenance.
4. Periodic inspection of stored equipment.
5. Periodic inspection when a question arises concerning the appropriateness of selected equipment, or when problems with similar equipment are discovered.

Each inspection will cover different areas with varying degrees of depth. Those personnel responsible for clothing inspection should follow manufacturer directions; many vendors provide detailed inspection procedures. The generic inspection checklist provided in Table VIII:1-7 may serve as an initial guide for developing more extensive procedures.

Records must be kept of all inspection procedures. Individual identification numbers should be assigned to all reusable pieces of equipment (many clothing and equipment items may already have serial numbers), and records should be maintained by that number. At a minimum, each inspection should record:

- Clothing/equipment item ID number;
- Date of the inspection;
- Person making the inspection;
- Results of the inspection; and
- Any unusual conditions noted.

Periodic review of these records can provide an indication of protective clothing which requires excessive maintenance and can also serve to identify clothing that is susceptible to failure.

TABLE VIII:1-7. SAMPLE PPE INSPECTION CHECKLISTS
Clothing

Before use:	Determine that the clothing material is correct for the specified task at hand.

Visually inspect for:

- Imperfect seams;
- Nonuniform coatings;
- Tears; and
- Malfunctioning closures.

Hold up to light and check for pinholes

Flex product:

- Observe for cracks.
- Observe for other signs or shelf deterioration.

If the product has been used previously, inspect inside and out for signs of chemical attack:

- Discoloration
- Swelling
- Stiffness

During the work task, periodically inspect for:

- Evidence of chemical attack such as discoloration, swelling, stiffening and softening.
- Keep in mind, however, that chemic permeation can occur without any vi effects.
- Closure failure
- Tears
- Punctures
- Seam discontinuities

Gloves

Before use:

Pressurize glove to check for pinholes. Either blow into glove, then roll gauntlet towards fingers or inflate glove and hold under water. In either case, no air should escape.

Fully Encapsulating Suits

Before use:

- Check the operation of pressure re[lief]
  valves
- Inspect the fitting of wrists, ankles,
- Check faceshield, if so equipped, fo[r]
  - cracks
  - crazing
  - fogginess

STORAGE.

Clothing must be stored properly to prevent damage or malfunction from exposure to dust, moisture, sunlight, damaging chemicals, extreme temperatures and impact. Procedures are needed for both initial receipt of equipment and after use or exposure of that equipment. Many manufacturers specify recommended procedures for storing their products. These should be followed to avoid equipment failure resulting from improper storage.

Some guidelines for general storage of chemical protective clothing include:

- Potentially contaminated clothing should be stored in an area separate from street clothing or unused protective clothing.
- Potentially contaminated clothing should be stored in a well-ventilated area, with good air flow around each item, if possible.
- Different types and materials of clothing and gloves should be stored separately to prevent issuing the wrong material by mistake (e.g. many glove materials are black and cannot be identified by appearance alone).
- Protective clothing should be folded or hung in accordance with manufacturer instructions.

MAINTENANCE.

Manufacturers frequently restrict the sale of certain protective suit parts to individuals or groups who are specially trained, equipped, or authorized by the manufacturer to purchase them. Explicit procedures should be adopted to ensure that the appropriate level of maintenance is performed only by those individuals who have this specialized training and equipment. In no case should you attempt to repair equipment without checking with the person in your facility who is responsible for chemical protective clothing maintenance.

The following classification scheme is recommended to divide the types of permissible or nonpermissible repairs:

- **Level 1:** User or wearer maintenance, requiring a few common tools or no tools at all.
- **Level 2:** Maintenance that can be performed by the response team's maintenance shop, if adequately equipped and trained.
- **Level 3** : Specialized maintenance that can be performed only by the factory or an authorized repair person.

Each facility should adopt the above scheme and list which repairs fall into each category for each type of protective clothing and equipment. Many manufacturers will also indicate which repairs, if performed in the field, void the warranty of their products. All repairs made must be recorded on the records for the specific clothing along with appropriate inspection results.

IX. TRAINING.

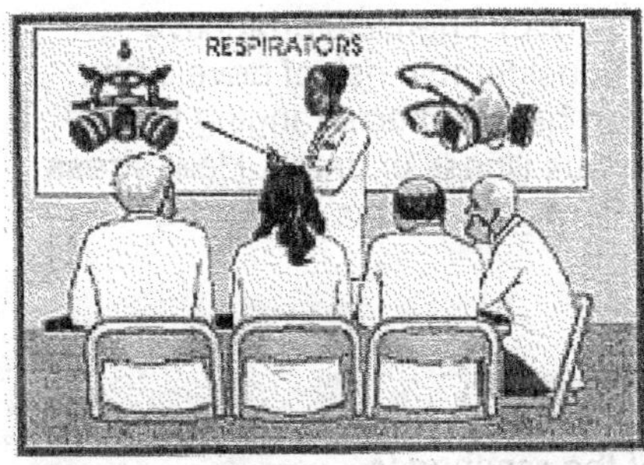

BENEFITS. Training in the use of protective clothing:

- Allows the user to become familiar with the equipment in a nonhazardous, nonemergency condition.
- Instills confidence of the user in his/her equipment.
- Makes the user aware of the limitations and capabilities of the equipment.
- Increases worker efficiency in performing various tasks.
- Reduces the likelihood of accidents during chemical operations.

CONTENT. Training should be completed prior to actual clothing use in a non-hazardous environment and should be repeated at the frequency required by OSHA SARA III legislation. As a minimum the training should point out the user's responsibilities and explain the following, using both classroom and field training when necessary, as follows:

- The proper use and maintenance of selected protective clothing, including capabilities and limitations.
- The nature of the hazards and the consequences of not using the protective clothing.
- The human factors influencing protective clothing performance.
- Instructions in inspecting, donning, checking, fitting, and using protective clothing.
- Use of protective clothing in normal air for a long familiarity period.
- The user's responsibility (if any) for decontamination, cleaning, maintenance, and repair of protective clothing.
- Emergency procedures and self-rescue in the event of protective clothing/ equipment failure.
- The buddy system.

The discomfort and inconvenience of wearing chemical protective clothing and equipment can create a resistance to its conscientious use. One essential aspect of training is to make the user aware of the need for protective clothing and to instill motivation for the proper use and maintenance of that protective clothing.

X. RISKS.

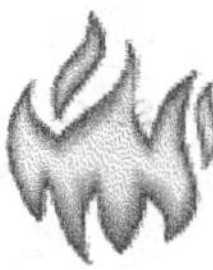

HEAT STRESS. Wearing full body chemical protective clothing puts the wearer at considerable risk of developing heat stress. This can result in health effects ranging from transient heat fatigue to serious illness or death. Heat stress is caused by a number of interacting factors, including:

- Environmental conditions;
- Type of protective ensemble worn;
- The work activity required; and
- The individual characteristics of the responder.

When selecting chemical protective clothing and equipment, each item's benefit should be carefully evaluated for its potential for increasing the risk of heat stress. For example, if a lighter, less insulating suit can be worn without a sacrifice in protection, then it should be. Because the incidence of heat stress depends on a variety of factors, all workers wearing full body chemical protective ensembles should be monitored.

The following physiological factors should be monitored.

HEART RATE. Count the radial pulse during a 30-second period as early as possible in any rest period. If the heart rate exceeds 110 beats per minute at the beginning of the rest period, the next work cycle should be shortened by one-third.

ORAL TEMPERATURE.

Do not permit an end user to wear protective clothing and engage in work when his or her oral temperature exceeds 100.6°F (38.1°C).

Use a clinical thermometer (three minutes under the tongue) or similar device to measure oral temperature at the end of the work period (before drinking), as follows:

- If the oral temperature exceeds 99.6°F (37.6°C), shorten the next work period by at least one-third.
- If the oral temperature exceeds 99.6°F (37.6°C) at the beginning of a response period, shorten the mission time by one-third.

BODY WATER LOSS. Measure the end user's weight on a scale accurate to plus or minus 0.25 pounds prior to any response activity. Compare this weight with his or her normal body weight to determine if enough fluids have been consumed to prevent dehydration. Weights should be taken while the end user wears similar clothing, or ideally, in the nude. The body water loss should not exceed 1.5% of the total body weight loss from a response.

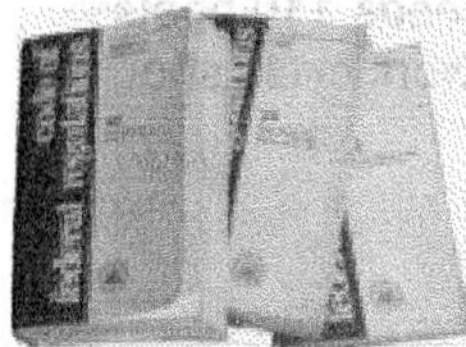

A complete copy of OSHA 29 CFR 1910.120 regulations [Hazardous Waste Operations and Emergency Response] is provided as a supplement to this course.

The Resource Conservation and Recovery Act (RCRA) mandated a cradle-to-grave system of managing hazardous waste. Regulations adopted by the Environmental Protection Agency (EPA) carry out the RCRA mandate. The chain of regulation extends to those who generate, transport, store, treat, and dispose of hazardous waste.

The EPA is not the only agency that regulates hazardous waste. Both the EPA and the Department of Transportation (DOT) regulate the transportation of hazardous waste. You will find references to the EPA regulations in the DOT regulations and vice versa.

The Occupational Safety and Health Administration (OSHA) issued a standard covering all workers employed in clean-up operations at uncontrolled hazardous waste sites and at EPA licensed TSD facilities. The standard covers workers responding to emergencies involving hazardous materials, spills. EPA and DOT also have regulations covering personnel training and emergency response.

1. Occupational Safety and Health Act - OSHA [1970]

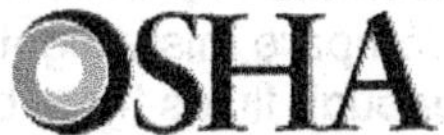

Congress passed the Occupational and Safety Health Act to ensure worker and workplace safety. Their Goal was to make sure employers provide their workers a place of employment free from recognized hazards to safety and health, such as exposure to toxic chemicals, excessive noise levels, mechanical dangers, heat or cold stress, or unsanitary conditions.

In order to establish standards for workplace health and safety, the Act also created the National Institute for Occupational Safety and Health (NIOSH) as the research institution for the Occupational Safety and Health Administration (OSHA). OSHA is a division of the U.S. Department of Labor that oversees the administration of the Act and enforces standards in all 50 states.

2. Environmental Protection Agency – EPA

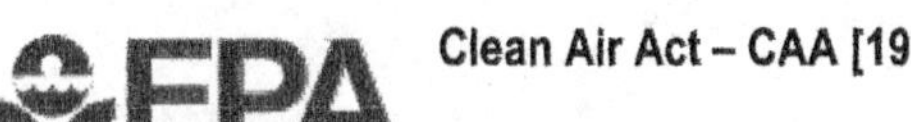

Clean Air Act – CAA [1970]

The Clean Air Act is the comprehensive Federal law that regulates air emissions from area, stationary, and mobile sources. This law authorizies the U.S. Environmental Protection Agency to establish National Ambient Air Quality Standards (NAAQS) to protect public health and the environment.

The goal of the Act was to set and achieve NAAQS in every state. The setting of maximum pollutant standards was coupled with directing the states to develop state implementation plans (SIP's) applicable to appropriate industrial sources in the state.

The Act was amended in 1977 primarily to set new goals (dates) for achieving attainment of NAAQS since many areas of the country had failed to meet the deadlines. Recently amendments to the Clean Air Act in large part were intended to meet unaddressed or insufficiently addressed problems such as acid rain, ground-level ozone, stratospheric ozone depletion, and air toxics.

Clean Water Act –CWA [1972]

Growing public awareness and concern for controlling water pollution led to enactment of the Federal Water Pollution Control Act Amendments of 1972. As amended in 1977, this law became commonly known as the Clean Water Act. The Act established the basic structure for regulating discharges of pollutants into the waters of the United States. It gave EPA the authority to implement pollution control programs such as setting wastewater standards for industry. The Clean Water Act also continued requirements to set water quality standards for all contaminants in surface waters. The Act made it unlawful for any person to discharge any pollutant from a point source into navigable waters, unless a permit was obtained under its provisions. It also funded the construction of sewage treatment plants under the construction grants program and recognized the need for planning to address the critical problems posed by nonpoint source pollution.

Subsequent enactments modified some of the earlier Clean Water Act provisions. Revisions in 1981 streamlined the municipal construction grants process, improving the capabilities of treatment plants built under the program. Changes in 1987 phased out the construction grants program, replacing it with the State Water Pollution Control Revolving Fund, more commonly known as the Clean Water State Revolving Fund. This new funding strategy addressed water quality needs by building on EPA-State partnerships.

Comprehensive Environmental Response, Compensation, and Liability Act (Superfund) – CERCLA [1980]

CERCLA (pronounced SIR-cla) provides a Federal "Superfund" to clean up uncontrolled or abandoned hazardous-waste sites as well as accidents, spills, and other emergency releases of pollutants and contaminants into the environment. Through the Act, EPA was given power to seek out those parties responsible for any release and assure their cooperation in the cleanup.

EPA cleans up orphan sites when potentially responsible parties cannot be identified or located, or when they fail to act. Through various enforcement tools, EPA obtains private party cleanup through orders, consent decrees, and other small party settlements. EPA also recovers costs from financially viable individuals and companies once a response action has been completed.

EPA is authorized to implement the Act in all 50 states and U.S. territories. Superfund site identification, monitoring, and response activities in states are coordinated through the state environmental protection or waste management agencies.

Emergency Planning & Community Right to Know Act – EPCRA [1986]

Also known as Title III of <u>SARA</u>, EPCRA was enacted by Congress as the national legislation on community safety. This law was designated to help local communities protect public health, safety, and the environment from chemical hazards.

To implement EPCRA, Congress required each state to appoint a State Emergency Response Commission (SERC). The SERC's were required to divide their states into Emergency Planning Districts and to name a Local Emergency Planning Committee (LEPC) for each district.

Broad representation by fire fighters, health officials, government and media representatives, community groups, industrial facilities, and emergency managers ensures that all necessary elements of the planning process are represented

Resource Conservation and Recovery Act –RCRA [1976]

Resource Conservation and Recovery Act - RCRA (pronounced "rick-rah") gave EPA the authority to control hazardous waste from the "cradle-to-grave." This includes the generation, transportation, treatment, storage, and disposal of hazardous waste. RCRA also set forth a framework for the management of non-hazardous wastes.

The 1986 amendments to RCRA enabled EPA to address environmental problems that could result from underground tanks storing petroleum and other hazardous substances. RCRA focuses only on active and future facilities and does not address abandoned or historical sites.

HSWA (pronounced "hiss-wa")—The Federal Hazardous and Solid Waste Amendments are the 1984 amendments to RCRA that required phasing out land disposal of hazardous waste. Some of the other mandates of this strict law include increased enforcement authority for EPA, more stringent hazardous waste management standards, and a comprehensive underground storage tank program.

Superfund Amendments and Reauthorization Act - [1986]

The Superfund Amendments and Reauthorization Act of 1986 reauthorized <u>CERCLA</u> to continue cleanup activities around the country. Several site-specific amendments, definitions clarifications, and technical requirements were added to the legislation, including additional enforcement authorities.

Title III of SARA also authorized the Emergency Planning and Community Right-to-Know Act

Toxic Substances Control Act – TSCA [1976]

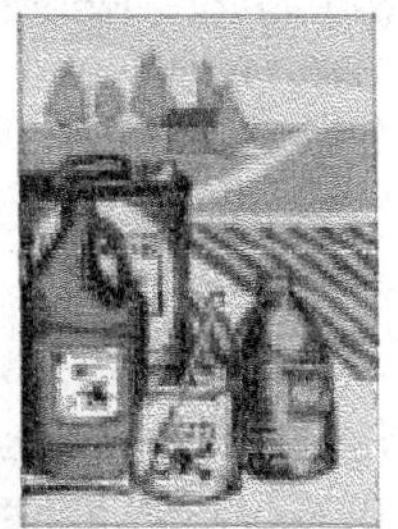

The Toxic Substances Control Act (TSCA) of 1976 was enacted by Congress to give EPA the ability to track the 75,000 industrial chemicals currently produced or imported into the United States. EPA repeatedly screens these chemicals and can require reporting or testing of those that may pose an environmental or human-health hazard. EPA can ban the manufacture and import of those chemicals that pose an unreasonable risk.

Also, EPA has mechanisms in place to track the thousands of new chemicals that industry develops each year with either unknown or dangerous characteristics. EPA then can control these chemicals as necessary to protect human health and the environment. TSCA supplements other Federal statutes, including the <u>Clean Air Act</u> and the Toxic Release Inventory under <u>EPCRA</u>

Chapter 10 -Summary 29CFR1910.120

The dumping of hazardous waste poses a significant threat to the environment. The Environmental Protection Agency's (EPA) 1995 data show that EPA managed about 277 million metric tons of hazardous waste at licensed *Resource Conservation and Recovery Act* (RCRA) sites. Hazardous waste is a serious safety and health problem that continues to endanger human and animal life and environmental quality. Hazardous Hazardous waste -- discarded chemicals that are toxic, flammable or corrosive -- can cause fires, explosions, and pollution of air, water, and land. Unless hazardous waste is properly treated, stored, or disposed of, it will continue to do great harm to all living things that come into contact with it now or in the future.

Because of the seriousness of the safety and health hazards related to hazardous waste operations, the Occupational Safety and Health Administration (OSHA) issued its **Hazardous Waste Operations and Emergency Response Standard, 29 C F R** 1910.120 to protect workers in this environment and to help them handle hazardous wastes safely and effectively.

State, county, and municipal employees such as police, ambulance workers, and firefighters with local fire departments will be covered by the regulations issued by the 25 states operating their own OSHA-approved safety and health programs (see listing at the end of this booklet). EPA regulations will cover these employees in states without state plans. These regulations will be based on OSHA's standard.

This summary discusses OSHA's requirements for hazardous waste operations and emergency response at uncontrolled hazardous waste sites and treatment, storage, and disposal (TSD) facilities and summarizes the steps an employer must take to protect the health and safety of workers in these environments.

Scope and Application

The standard covers workers in cleanup operations at uncontrolled hazardous waste sites and at EPA-licensed waste TSD facilities; as well as workers responding to emergencies involving hazardous materials (e.g., spills).

Provision of the Standard

Safety and Health Program

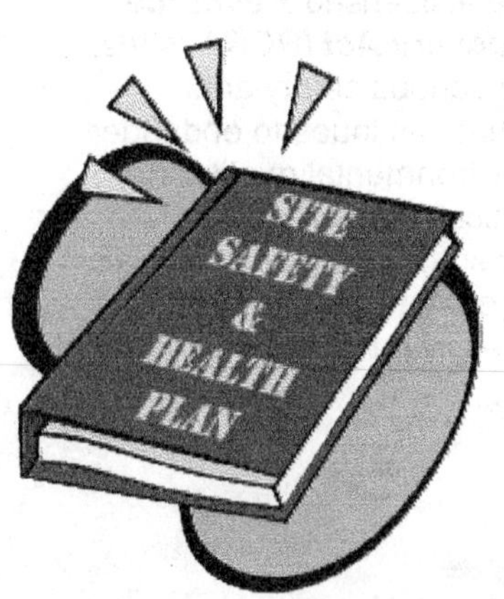

An effective and comprehensive safety and health program is essential in reducing work-related injuries and illnesses and in maintaining a safe and healthful work environment. The standard, therefore, requires each employer to develop and implement a written safety and health program that identifies, evaluates, and controls safety and health hazards and provides emergency response procedures for each hazardous waste site or treatment, storage, and disposal facility. This written program must include specific and detailed information on the following topics:

- An organizational workplan,
- Site evaluation and control,
- A site-specific program,
- Information and training program,
- Personal protective equipment program,
- Monitoring,
- Medical surveillance program,
- Decontamination procedures, and
- Emergency response program.

The written safety and health program must be periodically updated and made available to all affected employees, contractors, and subcontractors. The employer also must inform contractors and subcontractors, or their representatives, of any identifiable safety and health hazards or potential fire or explosion hazards before they enter the work site.

Each of the components of the safety and health program is discussed in the following paragraphs.

Workplan

Planning is the key element in a hazardous waste control program. Proper planning will greatly reduce worker hazards at waste sites. A workplan should support the overall objectives of the control program and provide procedures for implementation and should incorporate the employer's standard operating procedures for safety and health. Establishing a chain of command will specify employer and employee responsibilities in carrying out the safety and health program. For example, the plan should include the following:

- Supervisor and employee responsibilities and means of communication,
- Name of person who supervises all of the hazardous waste operations, and
- The site supervisor with responsibility for and authority to develop and implement the site safety and health program and to verify compliance.

In addition to this organizational structure, the plan should define the tasks and objectives of site operation as well as the logistics and resources required to fulfill these tasks. For example, the following topics should be addressed:

- The anticipated clean-up and/or operating procedures;
- A definition of work tasks and objectives and methods of accomplishment;
- The established personnel requirements for implementing the plan; and
- Procedures for implementing training, informational programs, and medical surveillance requirements.

Necessary coordination between the general program and site-specific activities also should be included in the actual operations workplan.

Site Evaluation and Control

Site evaluation, both initial and periodic, is crucial to the safety and health of workers. Site evaluation provides employers with the information needed to identify site hazards so they can select appropriate protection methods for employees.

It is extremely important, and a requirement of the standard, that a trained person conduct a preliminary evaluation of an uncontrolled hazardous waste site before entering the site. The evaluation must include all suspected conditions that are immediately dangerous to life or health or that may cause serious harm to employees (e.g., confined space entry, potentially explosive or flammable situations, visible vapor clouds, etc.). As available, the evaluation must include the location and size of the site, site topography, site accessibility by air and roads, pathways for hazardous substances to disperse, a description of worker duties, and the time needed to perform a given task, as well as the present status and capabilities of the emergency response teams.

Periodic reevaluations should also be conducted for treatment, storage, and disposal facilities, as conditions or operations change.

Controlling the activities of workers and the movement of equipment is an important aspect of the overall safety and health program. Effective control of the site will minimize potential contamination of workers, protect the public from hazards, and prevent vandalism. The following information is useful in implementing the site control program: a site map, site work zones, site communication, safe work practices, and the name, location and phone number of the nearest medical assistance.

The use of a "buddy system" also is required as a protective measure to assist in the rescue of an employee who becomes unconscious, trapped, or seriously disabled on site. In the buddy system, two employees must keep an eye on each other and only one should be in a specific dangerous area at one time, so that if one gets in trouble, the second can call for help.

Site-Specific Safety and Health Plan

A site-specific safety and health plan is a complementary program element that aids in eliminating or effectively controlling anticipated safety and health hazards. The site-specific plan must include all of the basic requirements of the overall safety and health program, but with attention to those characteristics unique to the particular site. For example, the site-specific plan may outline procedures for confined space entry, air and personal monitoring and environmental sampling, and a spill containment program to address the particular hazards present at the site.

The site safety and health plan must identify the hazards of each phase of the specific site operation and must be kept at the work site. Pre-entry briefings must be conducted prior to site entry and at other times as necessary to ensure that employees are aware of the site safety and health plan and its implementation. The employer also must ensure that periodic safety and health inspections are made of the site and that all known deficiencies are corrected prior to work at the site.

Information and Training Program

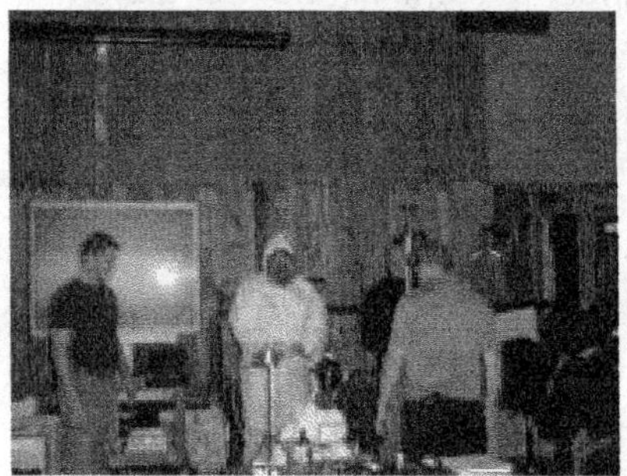

As part of the safety and health program, employers are required to develop and implement a program to inform workers (including contractors and subcontractors) performing hazardous waste operations of the level and degree of exposure they are likely to encounter.

Employers also are required to develop and implement procedures for introducing effective new technologies that provide improved worker protection in hazardous waste operations. Examples include foams, absorbents, adsorbents, and neutralizers.

Training makes workers aware of the potential hazards they may encounter and provides the necessary knowledge and skills to perform their work with minimal risk to their safety and health. The employer must develop a training program for all employees exposed to safety and health hazards during hazardous waste operations. Both supervisors and workers must be trained to recognize hazards and to prevent them; to select, care for and use respirators properly as well as other types of personal protective equipment; to understand engineering controls and their use; to use proper decontamination procedures; to understand the emergency response plan, medical surveillance requirements, confined space entry procedures, spill containment program, and any appropriate work practices. Workers also must know the names of personnel and their alternates responsible for site safety and health. The amount of instruction differs with the nature of the work operations, as indicated in Tables 1 and 2.

Employees at all sites must not perform any hazardous waste operations unless they have been trained to the level required by their job function and responsibility and have been certified by their instructor as having completed the necessary training. All emergency responders must receive refresher training, suffcient to maintain or demonstrate competency, annually. Employee training requirements are further defined by the nature of the work (e.g., temporary emergency response personnel, firefighters, safety officers, HAZMAT personnel, and incident commanders). These requirements may include recognizing and knowing the hazardous materials and their risks, knowing how to select and use appropriate personal protective equipment, and knowing the appropriate control, containment, or confinement procedures and how to implement them. The specific training and competency requirements for each personnel category are explained fully in the final rule For a brief summary of training requirements, see Tables 1 and 2.

Table 1. Training Requirements
Hazardous Waste Clean-Up Sites

Staff	
• Routine site employees	40 hours initial 24 hours field 8 hours annual refresher
• Routine site employees (minimal exposure)	24 hours initial 8 hours field 8 hours annual refresher
• Non-routine site employees	24 hours initial 8 hours field 8 hours annual refresher

Supervisors/Managers of	
• Routine site employees	40 hours initial 24 hours field 8 hours hazardous waste management 8 hours annual refresher
• Routine site employees (minimal exposure)	24 hours initial 8 hours field 8 hours hazardous waste management 8 hours annual refresher
• Non-routine site employees	24 hours initial 8 hours field 8 hours hazardous waste management 8 hours annual refresher

Treatment, Storage, and Disposal Sites Staff	
• General Site employees	24 hours initial or equivalent 8 hours annual refresher
• Emergency response personnel	Trained to a level of competency Annual refresher

Note: See 29 *CFR* 1910.120 (e) and (p)(7).

Table 2. Training Requirements

Other Emergency Response Staff	
Level 1 - First responder (awareness) level[1]	Sufficient training or proven experience in specific competencies Annual refresher
Level 2 - First responder (operations level)[2]	Level 1 competency and 8 hours initial or proven experience in specific competencies Annual refresher
Level 3 - HAZMAT technician[3]	24 hours of Level 2 and proven experience in specific competencies Annual refresher
Level 4 - HAZMAT specialist[4]	24 hours of Level 3 and proven experience in specific competencies Annual refresher
Level 5 - On-the-scene incident commander[5]	24 hours of Level 2 and additional competencies Annual refresher

Note: See 29 CFR 1910.120 (q) (6).

[1] Witnesses or discovers a release of hazardous materials and who are trained to notify the proper authorities.
[2] Responds to releases of hazardous substances in a defensive manner, without trying to stop the releases.
[3] Responds aggressively to stop the release of hazardous substances.
[4] Responds with and in support to HAZMAT technicians, but who have specific knowledge of various hazardous substances.
[5] Assumes control of the incident scene beyond the first-responder awareness level.

Employees who receive the training specified (see Table 1) must receive a written certificate upon successful completion of that training. That training need not be repeated if the employee goes to work at a new site; however, the employee must receive whatever additional training is needed to work safely at the new site. Employees who worked at hazardous waste sites before 1987 and received equivalent training need not repeat the initial training specified in Table 1, if the employer can demonstrate that in writing and certify that the employee has received such training.

Personal Protective Equipment Program

The standard further requires the employer to develop a written personal protective equipment program for all employees involved in hazardous waste operations. As mentioned earlier, this program also is part of the site-specific safety and health program. The personal protective

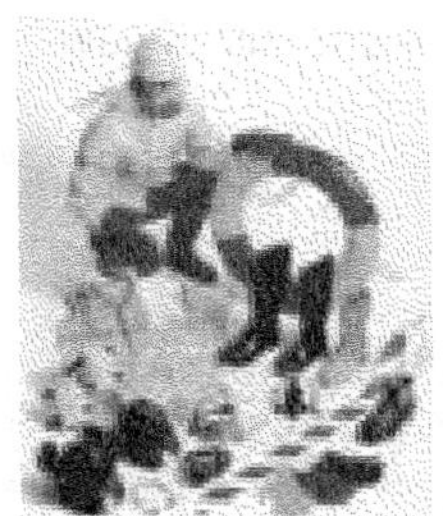

equipment program must include an explanation of equipment selection and use, maintenance and storage, decontamination and disposal, training and proper fit, donning and doffing procedures, inspection, in-use monitoring, program evaluation, and equipment limitations.

The employer also must provide and require the use of personal protective equipment where engineering control methods are infeasible to reduce worker exposures at or below the permissible exposure limit. Personal protective equipment must be selected that is appropriate to the requirements and limitations of the site, the task-specific conditions and duration, and the hazards and potential hazards identified at the site. As necessary, the employer must furnish the employee with positive-pressure self-contained breathing apparatus or positive-pressure air-line respirators equipped with an escape air supply, and with totally encapsulating chemical protective suits.

Monitoring

Airborne contaminants can present a significant threat to employee safety and health, thus making air monitoring an important component of 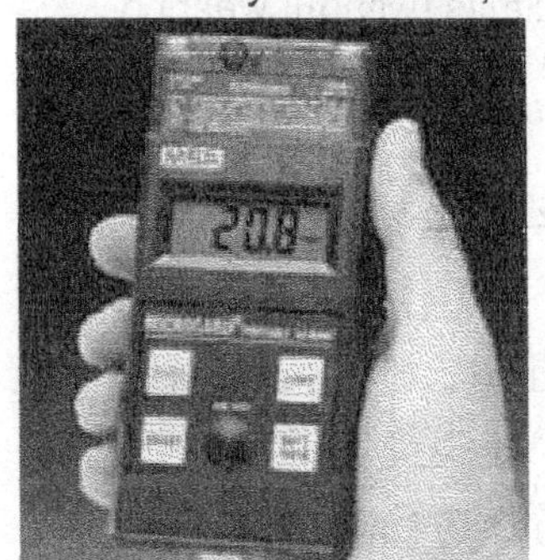 an effective safety and health program. The employer must conduct monitoring before site entry at uncontrolled hazardous waste sites to identify conditions immediately dangerous to life and health, such as oxygen-deficient atmospheres and areas where toxic substance exposures are above permissible limits. Accurate information on the identification and quantification of airborne contaminants is useful for the following:

- Selecting personal protective equipment,
- Delineating areas where protection and controls are needed,
- Assessing the potential health effects of exposure, and
- Determining the need for specific medical monitoring.

After a hazardous waste cleanup operation begins, the employer must periodically monitor those employees who are likely to have higher exposures to determine if they have been exposed to hazardous substances in excess of permissible exposure limits. The employer also must monitor for any potential condition that is immediately dangerous to life and health or for higher exposures that may occur as a result of new work operations.

Medical Surveillance

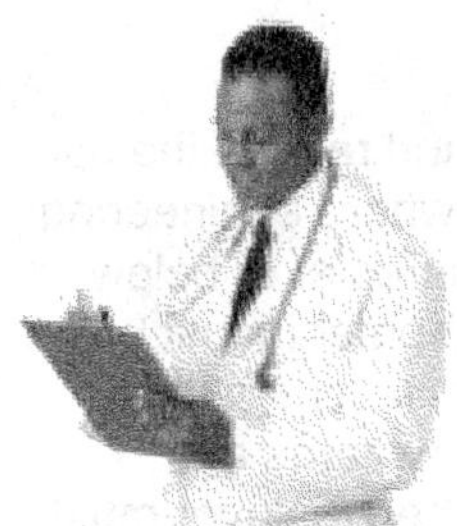

A medical surveillance program will help to assess and monitor the health and fitness of employees working with hazardous substances. The employer must establish a medical surveillance program for the following:

- All employees exposed or potentially exposed to hazardous substances or health hazards above permissible exposure limits for more than 30 days per year;
- Workers exposed above the published exposure levels (if there is no permissible exposure limit for these substances) for 30 days or more a year;
- Workers who wear approved respirators for 30 or more days per year on site;
- Workers who are exposed to unexpected or emergency releases of hazardous wastes above exposure limits (without wearing appropriate protective equipment) or who show signs, symptoms, or illness that may have resulted from exposure to hazardous substances; and
- Members of hazardous materials (HAZMAT) teams.

All examinations must be performed under the supervision of a licensed physician, without cost to the employee, without loss of pay and at a reasonable time and place. Examinations must include a medical and work history with special emphasis on symptoms related to the handling of hazardous substances and health hazards and to fitness for duty including the ability to wear any required personal protective equipment under conditions that may be expected at the work site. These examinations must be given as follows:

- Prior to job assignment and annually thereafter (or every 2 years if a physician determines that is sufficient),
- At the termination of employment,[2]
- Before reassignment to an area where medical examinations are not required,[2]
- If the examining physician believes that a periodic followup is medically necessary, and

- As soon as possible for employees injured or becoming ill from exposure to hazardous substances during an emergency, or who develop signs or symptoms of overexposure from hazardous substances.

The employer must give the examining physician a copy of the standard and its appendices, a description of the employee's duties relating to his or her exposure, the exposure level or anticipated exposure level, a description of any personal protective and respiratory equipment used or to be used, and any information from previous medical examinations. The employer must obtain a written opinion from the physician that contains the results of the medical examination and any detected medical conditions that would place the employee at an increased risk from exposure, any recommended limitations on the employee or upon the use of personal protective equipment, and a statement that the employee has been informed by the physician of the medical examination. The physician is not to reveal, in the written opinion given to the employer, specific findings or diagnoses unrelated to employment.

Decontamination Procedures

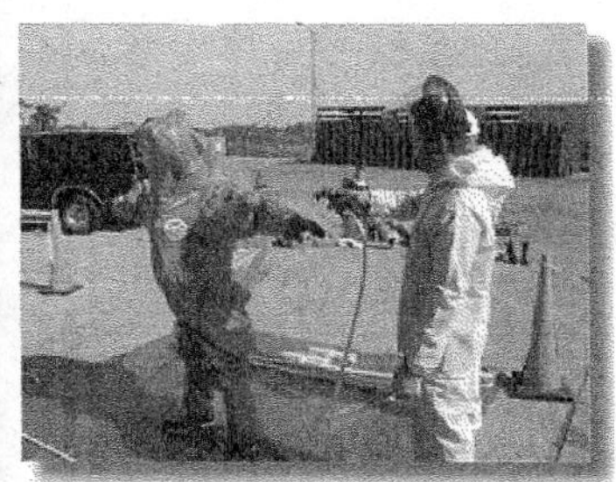

Decontamination procedures are a component of the site-specific safety and health plan and, consequently, must be developed, communicated to employees, and implemented before workers enter a hazardous waste site. As necessary, the site safety and health officer must require and monitor decontamination of the employee or decontamination and disposal of the employee's clothing and equipment, as well as the solvents used for decontamination, before the employee leaves the work area. If an employee's non-impermeable clothing becomes grossly contaminated with hazardous substances, the employee must immediately remove that clothing and take a shower. Impermeable protective clothing must be decontaminated before being removed by the employee.

Protective clothing and equipment must be decontaminated, cleaned, laundered, maintained, or replaced to retain effectiveness. The employer must inform any person who launders or cleans such clothing or equipment of the potentially harmful effects of exposure to hazardous substances.

Employees who are required to shower must be provided showers and change rooms that meet the requirements of 29 CFR 1910.141, *Subpart*

J -- General Environmental Controls. In addition, unauthorized employees must not remove their protective clothing or equipment from change rooms unless authorized to do so.

Emergency Response

Proper emergency planning and response are important elements of the safety and health program that help minimize employee exposure and injury. The standard requires that the employer develop and implement a written emergency response plan to handle possible emergencies before performing hazardous waste operations. The plan must include, at uncontrolled hazardous waste sites and at treatment, storage, and disposal facilities, the following elements:[3]

- Personnel roles, lines of authority, and communication procedures,
- Pre-emergency planning,
- Emergency recognition and prevention,
- Emergency medical and first-aid treatment,
- Methods or procedures for alerting onsite employees,
- Safe distances and places of refuge,
- Site security and control,
- Decontamination procedures,
- Critique of response and followup,
- Personal protective and emergency equipment, and
- Evacuation routes and procedures.

In addition to the above requirements, the plan must include site topography, layout, and prevailing weather conditions; and procedures for reporting incidents to local, state, and federal government agencies.

The procedures must be compatible with and integrated into the disaster, fire and/or emergency response plans of the site's nearest local, state, and federal agencies. Emergency response organizations may use the local or state emergency response plans, or both, as part of their emergency response plan to avoid duplication of federal regulations.

The plan requirements also must be rehearsed regularly, reviewed periodically, and amended, as necessary, to keep them current with new or changing site conditions or information. A distinguishable and distinct alarm system must be in operation to notify employees of emergencies. The emergency plan also must be made available for inspection and copying by employees, their representatives, OSHA personnel, and other governmental agencies with relevant responsibilities.

When deemed necessary, employees must wear positive-pressure self-contained breathing apparatus and approved self-contained compressed-air breathing apparatus with approved cylinders. In addition, back-up and first-aid support personnel must be available for assistance or rescue.

As already indicated, as part of an effective safety and health program, the employer must institute control methods and work practices that are appropriate to the specific characteristics of the site. Such controls are essential to successful worker protection. Some control methods are described in the following paragraphs.

Engineering Controls and Work Practices

To the extent feasible, the employer must institute engineering controls and work practices to help reduce and maintain employee exposure at or below permissible exposure limits. To the extent not feasible, engineering and work practice controls may be supplemented with personal protective equipment. Examples of suitable and feasible engineering controls include the use or pressurized cabs or control booths on equipment, and/or remotely operated materials handling equipment. Examples of safe work practices include removing all non-essential employees from potential exposure while opening drums, wetting down dusty operations, and placing employees upwind of potential hazards.

Handling and Labeling Drums and Containers

Prior to handling a drum or container, the employer must assure that
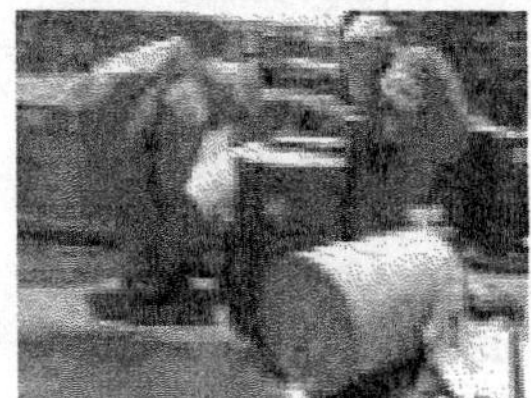
drums or containers meet the required OSHA, EPA (40 *CFR* Parts 264-265 and 300), and Department of Transportation (DOT) regulations (49 *CFR* Parts 171-178), and are properly inspected and labeled. Damaged drums or containers must be emptied of their contents, using a device classified for the material being transferred, and must be properly discarded. In areas where spills, leaks or ruptures occur, the employer must furnish employees with salvage drums or containers, a suitable quantity of absorbent material, and approved fire-extinguishing equipment in the event of small fires. The employer also must inform employees of the appropriate hazard warnings of labeled drums, the removal of soil or coverings, and the dangers of handling unlabeled drums or containers without prior

identification of their contents. To the extent feasible, the moving of drums or containers must be kept to a minimum, and a program must be implemented to contain and isolate hazardous substances being transferred into drums or containers. In addition, an approved EPA ground-penetrating device must be used to determine the location and depth of any improperly discarded drums or containers.

The employer also must ensure that safe work practices are instituted before opening a drum or container. For example, air-line respirators and approved electrical equipment must be protected from possible contamination, and all equipment must be kept behind any existing explosion barrier.

Only tools or equipment that prevent ignition shall be used. All employees not performing the operation shall be located at a safe distance and behind a suitable barrier to protect them from accidental explosions. In addition, standing on or working from drums or containers is prohibited. Special care also must be given when an employee handles containers of shock-sensitive waste, explosive materials, or laboratory waste packs. Where an emergency exists, the employer must ensure the following:

- Evacuate non-essential employees from the transfer area;
- Protect equipment operators from exploding containers by using a barrier, and
- Make available a continuous means of communication (e.g., suitable radios or telephones), and a distinguishable and distinct alarm system to signal the beginning and end of activities where explosive wastes are handled.

If drums or containers bulge or swell or show crystalline material on the outside, they must not be moved onto or from the site unless appropriate containment procedures have been implemented. In addition, lab packs must be opened only when necessary and only by a qualified person. Prior to shipment to a licensed disposal facility, all drums or containers must be properly labeled and packaged for shipment. Staging areas also must be kept to a minimum and provided with adequate access and egress routes.

Sanitation of Temporary Workplaces

Each temporary worksite must have a supply of potable water that is stored in tightly closed and clearly labelled containers and equipped with a tap. Disposable cups and a receptacle for cup disposal also must be provided. The employer also must clearly mark all water outlets that are unsafe for drinking, washing, or cooking. Temporary worksites must be equipped with toilet facilities. If there are no sanitary sewers close to or on the hazardous waste site, the employer must provide the following toilet facilities unless prohibited by local codes:

- Privies,
- Chemical toilets,
- Recirculating toilets, or
- Combustion toilets.

Heated, well-ventilated, and well-lighted sleeping quarters must be provided for workers who guard the worksite. In addition, washing facilities for all workers must be near the worksite, within controlled work zones, and so equipped to enable employees to remove hazardous substances. The employer also must ensure that food service facilities are licensed.

Recordkeeping

In 1988, OSHA revised the standard requiring employers to provide employees with information to assist in the management of their own safety and health. The standard, *Access to Employee Exposure and Medical Records* (29 CFR 1910.20), permits direct access to these records by employees exposed to hazardous materials, or by their designated representatives, and by OSHA. The rule applies to, but does not require, medical and exposure records maintained by the employer.

The employer must keep exposure records for 30 years and medical records for at least the duration of employment plus 30 years. Records of employees who have worked for less than 1 year need not be retained after employment, but the employer must provide these records to the employee upon termination of employment. First-aid records of one-time treatment need not be retained for any specified period.

The employer must inform each employee of the existence, location, and availability of these records. Whenever an employer plans to stop doing business and there is no successor employer to receive and maintain these records, the employer must notify employees of their right to access to records at least 3 months before the employer ceases to do business. At the same time, employers also must notify the National Institute for Occupational Safety and Health.

Under the hazardous waste standard, at a minimum, medical records must include the following information:

- Employee's name and social security number
- Physicians' written opinions,
- Employee's medical complaints related to exposure to hazardous substances, and
- Information provided to the treating physician.

Hazard Communication Standard (HAZCOM)

Title III of the *Superfund Amendments and Reauthorization Act of 1986* (SARA) requires employers covered by the *Hazard Communication Standard* (29 *CFR* 1910. 1200) to maintain Material Safety Data Sheets (MSDSs) and submit such information to State emergency response commissions, local emergency planning committees, and the local fire department. Under this requirement, employers covered by HCS must provide chemical hazard information to both employees and surrounding communities. Consequently, in the case of an emergency response situation to hazardous substances at a site, the local fire department may already be aware of the chemicals present at the site since data may have been provided through MSDSs

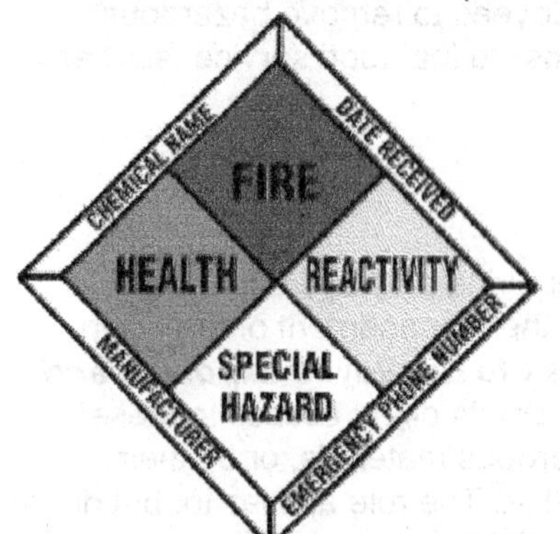

Appendix A- NIOSH Pocket Guide to Chemical Hazards

The *NIOSH Pocket Guide to Chemical Hazards* is intended as a source of general industrial hygiene information for workers, employers, and occupational health professionals. The *Pocket Guide* presents key information and data in abbreviated tabular form for 677 chemicals or substance groupings (e.g., manganese compounds, tellurium compounds, inorganic tin compounds, etc.) that are found in the work environment. The industrial hygiene information found in the *Pocket Guide* should help users recognize and control occupational chemical hazards. The chemicals or substances contained in this revision include all substances for which the National Institute for Occupational Safety and Health (NIOSH) has recommended exposure limits (RELs) and those with permissible exposure limits (PELs) as found in the Occupational Safety and Health Administration (OSHA) General Industry Air Contaminants Standard (29 CFR 1910.1000).

Background

In 1974, NIOSH (which is responsible for recommending health and safety standards) joined OSHA (whose jurisdictions include promulgation and enforcement activities) in developing a series of occupational health standards for substances with existing PELs. This joint effort was labeled the Standards Completion Program and involved the cooperative efforts of several contractors and personnel from various divisions within NIOSH and OSHA. The Standards Completion Program developed 380 substance-specific draft standards with supporting documentation that contained technical information and recommendations needed for the promulgation of new occupational health regulations. The *Pocket Guide* was developed to make the technical information in those draft standards more conveniently available to workers, employers, and occupational health professionals. The *Pocket Guide* is updated periodically to reflect new data regarding the toxicity of various substances and any changes in exposure standards or recommendations.

Data Collection and Application

The data were collected from a variety of sources, including NIOSH policy documents such as criteria documents and Current Intelligence Bulletins (CIBs), and recognized references in the fields of industrial hygiene, occupational medicine, toxicology, and analytical chemistry.

NIOSH RECOMMENDATIONS

Acting under the authority of the Occupational Safety and Health Act of 1970 (29 USC Chapter 15) and the Federal Mine Safety and Health Act of 1977 (30 USC Chapter 22), NIOSH develops and periodically revises recommended exposure limits (RELs) for hazardous substances or conditions in the workplace. NIOSH also recommends appropriate preventive measures to reduce or eliminate the adverse health and safety effects of these hazards. To formulate these recommendations, NIOSH evaluates all known and available medical, biological, engineering, chemical, trade, and other information relevant to the hazard. These recommendations are then published and transmitted to OSHA and the Mine Safety and Health Administration (MSHA) for use in promulgating legal standards.

Alerts, Special Hazard Reviews, Occupational Hazard Assessments, and Technical Guidelines support and complement the other standards development activities of the Institute. Their purpose is to assess the safety and health problems associated with a given agent or hazard (e.g., the potential for injury or for carcinogenic, mutagenic, or teratogenic effects) and to recommend appropriate control and surveillance methods. Although these documents are not intended to supplant the more comprehensive criteria documents, they are prepared to assist OSHA and MSHA in the formulation of regulations.

A complete list of occupational safety and health issues for which NIOSH has formal policies (e.g., recommendations for occupational exposure to chemical and physical hazards, engineering controls, work practices, safety considerations, etc.) can be found in *NIOSH Recommendations for Occupational Safety and Health: Compendium of Policy Documents and Statements* [DHHS (NIOSH) Publication No. 92-100].

HOW TO USE THIS POCKET GUIDE

The Pocket Guide has been designed to provide chemical-specific data to supplement general industrial hygiene knowledge. To maximize the amount of data provided in this limited space, abbreviations and codes have been used extensively. These abbreviations and codes, which have been designed to permit rapid comprehension by the regular user, are discussed for each column in the following subsections.

Chemical Name and Structure/Formula, CAS and RTECS Numbers, and DOT ID and Guide Numbers

Chemical Name and Structure/Formula - The chemical name found in the OSHA General Industry Air Contaminants Standard (29 CFR 1910.1000) is listed first. The chemical formula is also provided under the chemical name.

CAS and RTECS Numbers - The Chemical Abstracts Service (CAS) number, in the format xxx-xx-x, is unique for each chemical and allows efficient searching on computerized data bases. The *NIOSH Registry of Toxic Effects of Chemical Substances* (RTECS) number, in the format ABxxxxxxx, may be useful for obtaining additional toxicologic information on a specific substance.

DOT ID and GUIDE Number - The U.S. Department of Transportation (DOT) identification number and the corresponding guide number. Their format is xxxx xxx. The Identification number (xxxx) indicates that the chemical is regulated by DOT. The Guide number (xxx) refers to actions to be taken to stabilize an emergency situation; this information can be found in the *2000 Emergency Response Guidebook* .

Synonyms, Trade Names, and Conversion Factors

Common synonyms and trade names are listed alphabetically for each chemical. Factors for the conversion of ppm (parts of vapor or gas per million parts of contaminated air by volume) to mg/m^3 (milligrams of vapor or gas per cubic meter of contaminated air) at 25 °C and 1 atmosphere are listed for chemicals with exposure limits expressed in ppm.

Exposure Limits

The NIOSH recommended exposure limits (RELs) are listed first in this column. Unless noted otherwise, RELs are time-weighted average (TWA) concentrations for up to a 10-hour workday during a 40-hour workweek. A short-term exposure limit (STEL) is designated by "ST" preceding the value; unless noted otherwise, the STEL is a 15-minute TWA exposure that should not be exceeded at any time during a workday. A ceiling REL is designated by "C" preceding the value; unless noted otherwise, the ceiling value should not be exceeded at any time. Any substance that NIOSH considers to be a potential occupational carcinogen is designated by the notation "Ca".

The OSHA permissible exposure limits (PELs), as found in Tables Z-1, Z-2, and Z-3 of the OSHA General Industry Air Contaminants Standard (29 CFR 1910.1000), that were effective on July 1, 1993[*] and which are

currently enforced by OSHA are listed next. [Note: In July 1992, the 11th
Circuit Court of Appeals in its decision in AFL-CIO v. OSHA, 965 F.2d
962 (11th Cir., 1992) vacated more protective PELs set by OSHA in
1989 for 212 substances, moving them back to PELs established in
1971. The appeals court also vacated new PELs for 164 substances that
were not previously regulated. The substances for which OSHA PELs
were vacated on June 30, 1993 are indicated by the symbol "†" following
OSHA PEL in this column. A number of RELs are based on NIOSH
concurrence with the data presented and the airborne exposure limits
proposed in this rulemaking.] Unless noted otherwise, PELs are TWA
concentrations that must not be exceeded during any 8-hour workshift of
a 40-hour workweek. A STEL is designated by "ST" preceding the value
and is measured over a 15-minute period unless noted otherwise. OSHA
ceiling concentrations (designated by "C" preceding the value) must not
be exceeded during any part of the workday; if instantaneous monitoring
is not feasible, the ceiling must be assessed as a 15-minute TWA
exposure. In addition, there are a number of substances from Table Z-2
(e.g., beryllium, ethylene dibromide, etc.) that have PEL ceiling values
that must not be exceeded except for specified excursions. For example,
a "5-minute maximum peak in any 2 hours" means that a 5-minute
exposure above the ceiling value, but never above the maximum peak, is
allowed in any 2 hours during an 8-hour workday.

Concentrations are given in ppm, mg/m^3, mppcf (millions of particles per
cubic foot of air as determined from counting an impinger sample), or
fibers/cm^3 (fibers per cubic centimeter). The "[skin]" designation indicates
the potential for dermal absorption; skin exposure should be prevented
as necessary through the use of good work practices and gloves,
coveralls, goggles, and other appropriate equipment. The "(total)"
designation indicates that the REL or PEL listed is for "total particulate"
versus the "(resp)" designation which refers to the "respirable fraction" of
the airborne particulate.

IDLH

For the June 1994 Edition of the *Pocket Guide*, immediately dangerous
to life or health concentrations (IDLHs) were reviewed and, in many
cases, were revised and made more protective. As a consequence of the
IDLH changes, many of the respirator recommendations for these
substances were also revised. The criteria utilized to determine the
adequacy of existing IDLH values were a combination of those used
during the Standards Completion Program and a newer methodology
developed by NIOSH. These "interim" criteria form a tiered approach with
acute human toxicity data being used preferentially, followed next by
acute animal inhalation toxicity data, and then finally by acute animal oral

toxicity data to determine an updated IDLH value. When relevant acute toxicity data were insufficient or unavailable, the use of chronic toxicity data or an analogy to a chemically similar substance was considered. The criteria and information sources for both the original and revised IDLH values are given in _Documentation for Immediately Dangerous to Life and Health Concentrations (IDLHs)_ (NTIS Publication No. PB-94-195047). NIOSH is currently assessing the various uses of IDLHs and whether the original criteria used to derive the IDLH values are valid or if other information or criteria should be utilized. Based on this assessment, NIOSH will develop a new strategy for revising the IDLH values currently listed, as well as for developing new IDLH values for the more than 300 substances listed in the _Pocket Guide_ without IDLHs.

The definition of IDLH that was derived during the Standards Completion Program was based on the Mine Safety and Health Administration (MSHA) definition stipulated in 30 CFR 11.3(t). The purpose for establishing an IDLH value in the Standards Completion Program was to ensure that a worker could escape without injury or irreversible health effects from an IDLH exposure in the event of the failure of respiratory protection equipment. The IDLH was considered a maximum concentration above which only a highly reliable breathing apparatus providing maximum worker protection was permitted. In determining IDLH values, the ability of a worker to escape without loss of life or irreversible health effects was considered along with severe eye or respiratory irritation and other deleterious effects (e.g., disorientation or incoordination) that could prevent escape. As a safety margin, the Standards Completion Program IDLH values were based on the effects that might occur as a consequence of a 30-minute exposure. However, the 30-minute period was NOT meant to imply that workers should stay in the work environment any longer than necessary, in fact, EVERY EFFORT SHOULD BE MADE TO EXIT IMMEDIATELY!

The current NIOSH definition for an IDLH exposure condition, as stipulated in the _NIOSH Respirator Decision Logic_ [NIOSH] Publication No. 87-108, NTIS Publication No. PB-91-151183), is a condition "that poses a threat of exposure to airborne contaminants when that exposure is likely to cause death or immediate or delayed permanent adverse health effects or prevent escape from such an environment." The purpose of establishing an IDLH exposure concentration is to "ensure that the worker can escape from a given contaminated environment in the event of failure of the respiratory protection equipment." The _NIOSH Respirator Decision Logic_ uses these IDLH values as one of several respirator selection criteria. Under the _NIOSH Respirator Decision Logic_, the most protective respirators (e.g., a self-contained breathing apparatus equipped with a full facepiece and operated in a pressure-demand or other positive-pressure mode) would be selected for firefighting, exposure to carcinogens, entry into oxygen-deficient atmospheres, in emergency situations, during entry into an atmosphere that contains a substance at a concentration greater than 2,000 times the NIOSH REL or OSHA PEL, and for entry into IDLH atmospheres.

IDLH values are listed for over 380 substances. The notation "Ca" appears in this column for all substances that NIOSH considers to be potential occupational carcinogens. However, IDLH values that were originally determined in the Standards Completion Program or were recently revised are shown in brackets following the "Ca" designations. "10%LEL" indicates that the IDLH was based on 10% of the lower explosive limit for safety considerations even though the relevant toxicological data indicated that irreversible health effects or impairment of escape existed only at higher concentrations. "N.D." indicates that an IDLH has not as yet been determined.

Physical Description

This entry provides a brief description of the appearance and odor of each substance. Notations are made as to whether a substance can be shipped as a liquefied compressed gas or whether it has major use as a pesticide.

Chemical and Physical Properties

The following abbreviations are used for the chemical and physical properties given for each substance. "NA" indicates that a property is not applicable, and a question mark (?) indicates that it is unknown.

MW   Molecular weight

BP   Boiling point at 1 atmosphere, °F

Sol   Solubility in water at 68 °F (unless a different temperature is noted), % by weight (i.e., g/100 ml)

Fl.P   Flash point (i.e., the temperature at which the liquid phase gives off enough vapor to flash when exposed to an external ignition source), closed cup (unless annotated "(oc)" for open cup), °F

IP   Ionization potential, eV (electron volts) [Ionization potentials are given as a guideline for the selection of photoionization detector lamps used in some direct-reading instruments.]

VP   Vapor pressure at 68 °F (unless a different temperature is noted), mm Hg; "approx" indicates approximately

MLT   Melting point for solids, °F

FRZ   Freezing point for liquids and gases, °F

UEL   Upper explosive (flammable) limit in air, % by volume (at room temperature unless otherwise noted)

LEL   Lower explosive (flammable) limit in air, % by volume (at room temperature unless otherwise noted)

MEC   Minimum explosive concentration, g/m^3 (when available)

Sp.Gr   Specific gravity at 68 °F (unless a different temperature is noted) referenced to water at 39.2 °F (4 °C)

RGasD   Relative density of gases referenced to air = 1 (indicates how many times a gas is heavier than air at the same temperature)

When possible, the flammability/combustibility of a substance was determined and listed after the specific gravity. The following OSHA criteria (29 CFR 1910.106) were used to classify flammable or combustible liquids:

Class IA flammable liquid	Fl.P. below 73 °F and BP below 100 °F.
Class IB flammable liquid	Fl.P. below 73 °F and BP at or above 100 °F.
Class IC flammable liquid	Fl.P. at or above 73 °F and below 100 °F.
Class II combustible liquid	Fl.P. at or above 100 °F and below 140 °F.
Class IIIA combustible liquid	Fl.P. at or above 140 °F and below 200 °F.
Class IIIB combustible liquid	Fl.P. at or above 200 °F.

Incompatibilities and Reactivities

This entry lists important hazardous incompatibilities or reactivities of each substance.

Measurement Method

This entry provides a brief, key word description of the suggested sampling and analysis method. Each description comprises four components: (1) the collection method, (2) the sample work-up, (3) the analytical method, and (4) the method number. The method number is usually from the 4th edition of the *NIOSH Manual of Analytical Methods* (DHHS [NIOSH] Publication No. 94-113) and is indicated by "IV" following the sample work-up.

Personal Protection and Sanitation

This column presents a summary of recommended practices for each toxic substance. These recommendations supplement general work practices (e.g., no eating, drinking, or smoking where chemicals are used). Table 3 explains the codes used. Each category is described as follows:

SKIN: Recommends the need for personal protective clothing.

EYES: Recommends the need for eye protection.

WASH SKIN: Recommends when workers should wash the spilled chemical from the body in addition to normal washing (e.g., before eating).

REMOVE: Advises workers when to remove clothing that has accidentally become wet or significantly contaminated.

CHANGE: Recommends whether the routine changing of clothing is needed.

PROVIDE: Recommends the need for eyewash fountains and/or quick drench facilities.

First Aid

This entry lists <u>emergency procedures</u> for eye and skin contact, inhalation, and ingestion of the toxic substance.

Respirator Recommendations

This entry provides a condensed table of allowable respirator use for those substances for which IDLH values have been determined. NIOSH is currently reevaluating the IDLH values, and as new or revised IDLH values are developed, respirator selection recommendations will be incorporated into subsequent editions of the *Pocket Guide*. In the interim no respirator recommendations will be made for substances without IDLH values (these will be noted by "To be added later").

NIOSH has developed a new set of regulations in <u>42 CFR 84</u> (also referred to as "Part 84") for testing and certifying nonpowered, air-purifying, particulate-filter respirators. The new Part 84 respirators have passed a more demanding certification test than the old respirators (e.g.; dust; dust and mist; dust, mist, and fume; spray paint; pesticide; etc.) certified under 30 CFR 11 (also referred to as "Part 11"). Under Part 84, NIOSH is allowing manufacturers to continue selling and shipping Part 11 particulate filters as NIOSH-certified until July 10, 1998. It is important to see the <u>*NIOSH Guide to the Selection and Use of Particulate Respirators*</u> (DHHS [NIOSH] publication 96-101) for substitution of Part 84 respirators for Part 11 respirators.

The first line in the entry indicates whether the "NIOSH" or the "OSHA" exposure limit is used on which to base the respirator recommendations. The more protective limit between the NIOSH REL or the OSHA PEL is always used. "NIOSH/OSHA" indicates that the limits are equivalent.

Each subsequent line lists a maximum use concentration (MUC) followed by the classes of respirators, with their assigned protection factors (APFs), that are acceptable for use up to the MUC. Individual respirator classes are separated by diagonal lines (/). More protective respirators may be worn. Emergency or planned entry into unknown concentrations or entry into IDLH conditions are followed by the classes of respirators acceptable for these conditions. "Escape" indicates that the respirators are to be used only for escape purposes. For each MUC or condition this entry lists only those respirators with the required APF and other use restrictions based on the <u>*NIOSH Respirator Decision Logic*</u>.

In certain cases, the recommended respirators are annotated with the following symbols as additonal information:

* Substance reported to cause eye irritation or damage; may require eye protection

£ Substance causes eye irritation or damage; eye protection needed</TD< tr>

^ If not present as a fume

¿ Only nonoxidizable sorbents allowed (not charcoal)

† End of service life indicator (ESLI) required

All respirators selected must be approved by NIOSH and MSHA under the provisions of 30 CFR 11 or by NIOSH under <u>42 CFR 84</u>. The current listing of NIOSH certified respirators can be found in the *NIOSH Certified Equipment List* (DHHS [NIOSH] Publication No. 94-104)..

A complete respiratory protection program must be implemented and must fulfill all requirements of 29 CFR 1910.134. A respiratory protection program must include a written standard operating procedure covering regular training, fit-testing, fit-checking, periodic environmental monitoring, maintenance, medical monitoring, inspection, cleaning, storage and periodic program evaluation. Selection of a specific respirator within a given class of recommended respirators depends on the particular situation; this choice should be made only by a knowledgeable person. *REMEMBER:* Air-purifying respirators will not protect users against oxygen-deficient atmospheres, and they are not to be used in IDLH conditions. The only respirators recommended for fire fighting are self-contained breathing apparatuses that have full facepieces and are operated in a pressure-demand or other positive-pressure modes. Additional information on the selection and use of respirators can be found in the *NIOSH Respirator Decision Logic* and the *NIOSH Guide to Industrial Respiratory Protection* (DHHS [NIOSH] Publication No. 87-116).

Route of Health Hazard

This entry lists the toxicologically important routes of entry for each substance and whether contact with the skin or eyes is potentially hazardous.

Symptoms

This entry lists the potential symptoms of exposure.

Target Organs

This entry lists the organs that are affected by exposure to each substance.

Acid -a solution that has a pH value lower than

Acute- occurring only once or more than once within a short period of time

Acute Exposure -a single exposure to a hazardous material for a brief l length of time

Adverse Health Effect -any effect resulting in anatomical, functional, or psychological impairment that may affect the performance of the whole organism

Aquifer -an underground rock formation composed of sand, soil, gravel, or porous rock that can store and supply groundwater to wells and springs

Aquitard -a barrier to the flow of groundwater in an aquifer Assessment- see site assessment

Base -a solution that has a pH value greater than 7

Benthic -relating to or occurring at the bottom of a body of water

Biochemical Response -measure of a change in or damage to the blood chemistry of a species as a result of exposure to a contaminant

Biological Degradation -as used in the Superfund Program, the process by which biological agents can reduce or eliminate risks posed bya hazardous substance through decomposition into less hazardous components

Biomass -the amount of living matter in a given area, often refers to vegetation

Blood Enzyme Level -measure of a change in the enzymes normally present in the blood of a species as a result of exposure to a contaminant

Carcinogen -a substance or agent that may produce or increase the risk of cancer

Chronic Exposure -continuous or repeated exposure to a hazardous substance over a long period of time

Clay Soil -soil composed chiefly of fine particles

Clean Air Act- gives EPA authority to set standards for air quality and to control the release of airborne chemicals from industries, power plants, and cars

Cleanup -the process of removing, treating, or disposing of contaminants at a site and restoring the site to a condition that is not dangerous to people or the environment

Clean Water Act- a Federal law that controls the discharge of pollutants into surface water in a number of ways, including discharge permits

Community Involvement -a process in which the concerns of local citizens are addressed during the Superfund process

Composting -the decomposition of yard waste and vegetable scraps into organic material

Comprehensive Environmental Response, Compensation, and Liability Act (CERCLA) -enacted in 1980 and nicknamed Superfund, this law provides the authority through which the Federal government can compel people or companies responsible for creating hazardous waste sites to clean them up. It also created a public trust fund, known as the Superfund, to assist with the cleanup of inactive and abandoned hazardous waste sites or accidentally spilled or illegally dumped hazardous materials.

Concentration -the amount of one material dispersed or distributed in a larger amount of another material

Condensation -a part of the hydrologic cycle during which water vapor turns into a liquid

Confined Aquifer- an aquifer bounded on the top by confining materials such as rock formations

Contaminant- harmful or hazardous matter introduced into the environment Contaminant Level -a measure of how much of a contaminant is present

Contamination -the introduction of harmful or hazardous matter into the environment Corrective Action -cleanup of hazardous waste contamination at non-Superfund sites

Corrosive -capable of chemically wearing substances away (corroding) or destroying them

Deep-Well Injection- injection of hazardous wastes into deep wells underground

Dense Non-Aqueous Phase Liquid (DNAPL) -liquid contaminants that are relatively insoluble and heavier than water; also known as "sinkers" because they will sink to the bottom of an aquifer, where they become especially difficult to detect and clean up

Discharge Areas -locations where groundwater flows or is discharged to the surface

Discovery -the initial activity in the Superfund process where a potentially contaminated site is reported to EPA or a similar state or local agency

Diversity -variety; differences among and within species

Early Action -a response action that addresses the release or possible release of hazardous substances and can be resolved within a short period of time

Ecology- study of the relationships of living organisms to each other and to their environment

Ecosystem -a specialized community, including all the component organisms, that forms an interacting system; for example, a marsh, a shoreline, a forest

Emergency- a situation or occurrence of a serious nature that develops suddenly and unexpectedly and demands immediate action

Emergency Response -a response action to situations that may cause immediate and serious harm to people or the environment

Environment- totality of conditions surrounding an organism
Environmental Risk -likelihood, or probability, of injury, disease, or
death resulting from exposure to a potential environmental hazard
Epidemiology -study of causes of disease or toxic effects in human
populations --
Evaporation -a part of the hydrologic cycle during which liquid water
turns into water vapor
Exposure -coming into contact with a substance through inhalation,
ingestion, or direct contact with the skin; may be acute or chronic
Fauna- animal life
Federal Insecticide, Fungicide, and Rodenticide Act (FIFRA) -a
Federal law that requires labels on pesticides that provide clear
directions for safe use; FIFRA also authorizes EPA to set standards to
control how pesticides are used
Fertilizers- nitrogen- and phosphate-rich chemical compounds that are
used to increase the productivity of croplands; fertilizer production
usually includes the use and disposal of petrochemicals
Flora- plant life
Habitat Encroachment -term used to describe the way natural habitats
are destroyed as human development of new areas continues to grow
and expand, or pollution damages the environment
Hazard Ranking System (HRS) -the method EPA uses to assess and
score the hazards posed by a site that takes into account the nature and
extent of contamination and the potential for the hazardous substances
to migrate from the site through air, soil, surface water, or groundwater;
HRS scores are used to determine whether a site should be placed on
the National Priorities List (NPL)
Hazardous Chemical -see Hazardous Substance Hazardous Material -
see Hazardous Substance
Hazardous Substance -a broad term that includes all substances that
can be harmful to people or the environment; toxic substances,
hazardous materials and other similar terms are subsets of hazardous
substances
Hazardous Waste -by-products or waste materials of manufacturing and
other processes that have some dangerous property; generally
categorized as corrosive, ignitable, toxic, or reactive, or in some way
harmful to people or the environment
Health Risk Assessment -scientific evaluation of the probability of harm
resulting from exposure to hazardous materials
Heavy Metals -metals such as lead, chromium, copper, and cobalt that
can be toxic at relatively low concentrations
Histopathological Test -test that examines the structure of cells and
tissues to determine if any damage has been caused by exposure to a
contaminant
Hydrologic Cycle -the process of evaporation, transpiration,
condensation, precipitation, infiltration, runoff, and percolation in which

water molecules travel above, below, and on the Earth's surface

Ignitable- capable of bursting into flames easily

Infiltration -the movement of water through the ground surface into the unsaturated zone

Information Repository -a set of current information, technical reports, and reference documents regarding a Superfund site; it should be located in a public building that is convenient for local residents, such as a public school, city hall, or public library

Innovative Treatment Technologies -remedies that have been tested, selected, or used for treating hazardous waste or contaminated materials but don't have much information on cost and performance

Inorganic Compounds -chemical compounds that do not contain carbon, usually associated with life processes; for example, metals are inorganic

Landfill -a location for the disposal of wastes on land designed to protect the public from hazards in waste streams; **sanitary landfills,** designed to receive municipal solid waste, are distinguished from **hazardous waste landfills,** designed to isolate hazardous substances

Liability- under Superfund, a party responsible for the presence of hazardous waste at a site is also legally responsible for acting and paying to reduce or eliminate the risks posed by the site

Long- Term Action -a response action that eliminates or reduces a release or threatened release of hazardous substances that is serious but not an immediate danger to people or the environment and may take years to complete (also known as a remedial action)

Migration -as used in the Superfund program, the movement of a contaminant; actual or potential migration is one measure of the dangers created by a contaminant

Migration Pathways -the routes a contaminant may move around in the environment *(e.g.,* soil, groundwater, surface water, air)

Municipal Solid Waste- garbage that is disposed of in a sanitary or municipal solid waste landfill

Mutagenic -causing alteration in the DNA (genes or chromosomes) of an organism

National Priorities List (NPL) -EPA's list of the most serious uncontrolled or abandoned hazardous waste sites, identified as candidates for long-term action using money from the Superfund trust fund

Organic Compounds -chemical compounds that contain carbon, an element usually associated with life processes

Percolation -the movement of groundwater from the unsaturated zone to the saturated zone

Permeability -the degree to which groundwater can move freely through an aquifer measured by the interconnection of pores and fractures

Pesticides -chemical compounds used to control insects and other organisms that may reduce agricultural productivity; most are toxic

Appendix B 10 - Glossary

pH -a measurement of the acidity or alkalinity level of a solution
Physiological Response- measure of physical change or damage in a species as a result of exposure to a contaminant
Plume- an area of groundwater contamination
Pollution Prevention -a strategy that emphasizes reducing the amount of pollution or waste created, rather than controlling waste or dealing with pollutants after they have been created
Population -group of similar individuals living in the same general area
Pore -an open space in rocks and soils
Porosity- the ability of rock material to store water
Potentially Responsible Parties (PRPs) -any individual or company potentially responsible for, or contributing to, contamination at a Superfund site
Precipitation -a part of the hydrologic cycle during which condensed water vapor in the air falls to the ground in the form of rain, snow, sleet, and so forth
Preliminary Assessment (PA) -the process of collecting and reviewing available information about a known or suspected hazardous waste site or release that is used to determine if the site requires further study
Probability -chance that a given event will occur
Proposed Plan -a plan for cleaning up a Superfund site submitted by EPA and subject to public comments
Ratio -the relationship in quantity, amount, or size between two or more things
Reactive -one of four categories of hazardous waste; substances capable of changing into something else in the presence of other chemicals, usually violently or producing a hazardous by-product
Recharge Areas -areas where infiltration to aquifers occurs
Record of Decision (ROD) -a public document that explains the cleanup method that will be used at a Superfund site, based on EPA studies, public comments, and community concerns
Recycling -the reuse of products or by-products or other materials that could become wastes if discarded instead of being used
Relative Abundances -measure of the population of one species in an ecosystem as compared to other species within that same ecosystem; number of individuals in any given species compared to the total number of individuals in the community
Release -when a hazardous substance goes from a controlled condition (for example, inside a truck, barrel, storage tank, or landfill) to an uncontrolled condition in the air, water, or land
Residual Contamination -contaminants left at a site after the risks posed by the site have been reduced and the site no longer threatens people or the environment, or that currently is not possible to remove
Resource Conservation and Recovery Act (RCRA) -a Federal law that authorizes EPA to set standards for companies producing, handling, transporting, storing, and disposing of hazardous waste

Response Action -an action taken by EPA or another Federal, state, or local agency to address the risks posed by the release or threatened release of hazardous substances -generally categorized as Emergency Responses, Early Actions, and Long- Term Actions

Responsible Party -a person or business that is responsible for a hazardous site; whenever possible, EPA requires Responsible Parties, through administrative and legal actions, to clean up the sites they have contaminated

Risk -likelihood or probability of injury, disease, or death

Runoff -the amount of precipitation that runs over the ground surface and returns to streams, rivers, or other surface water bodies. It can collect pollutants from air or land and carry them to receiving waters

Safe Drinking Water Act (SDWA) -a Federal law that authorizes EPA to set national standards for drinking water and gives EPA authority to control the disposal of hazardous waste into groundwater

Sampling -the collection of representative specimens analyzed to characterize site conditions

Saturated Zone -an underground geologic layer in which all pores and fractures are filled with water

Saturation -the degree to which a geologic formation is filled with water

Site Assessment -the process by which EPA determines whether a potential Superfund site should be placed on the National Priorities List (NPL); it can consist of a Preliminary Assessment (PA) or a combination of a PA and a Site Inspection (SI)

Site Cleanup -see Cleanup

Site Discovery -see Discovery

Site Inspection (SI) -a technical phase of the Superfund process, following the Preliminary Assessment (PA), during which EPA gathers information (including sampling data) from a site needed to score the site using the Hazard Ranking System (HRS) to determine whether the site should be placed on the National Priorities List (NPL)

Solvents -chemical products that are used to dissolve other compounds; typically found in cleaners and used in petrochemical processes

Sorption -a process in which something is taken up and held; as used in the Superfund Program, sorption refers to technologies that use a sorption agent that attracts, takes up, and holds hazardous waste for removal

Source Reduction -the design, manufacture, or use of products that in some way reduces the amount of waste that must be disposed of; examples include reuse of by- products, reducing consumption, extending the useful life of a product, and minimizing materials going into production

Source Separation -the segregation of hazardous materials from nonhazardous materials to reduce the volume of hazardous waste that must meet special removal and disposal requirements; it is a method used by industry to control costs

Species Richness -number of species in a community Superfund -see CERCLA

Superfund Trust Fund -a public trust fund created with passage of the Comprehensive Environmental Response, Compensation, and Liability Act (CERCLA) in 1980 to be used to help pay for the cleanup of abandoned hazardous waste sites

Surface Impoundments -lined ponds storing hazardous waste

Surface Water -bodies of water that form and remain above ground, such as lakes, ponds, rivers, streams, bays, and oceans

Technical Assistance Grant (TAG) -funds given to communities for the purpose of hiring advisors to interpret technical information related to the cleanup of Superfund sites

Toxic- poisonous

Toxic Substances Control Act (TSCA) -a Federal law that empowers EPA to require the chemical industry to test chemicals and provide safety information before they are sold

Toxicology -study of the effects of poisons in living organisms

Transpiration -a part of the hydrologic cycle in which water vapor passes out of living organisms through a membrane or pores

Treatment Technologies -processes applied to hazardous waste or contaminated materials, to permanently alter their condition through chemical, biological, or physical means, and reduce or eliminate their danger to people and the environment

Unconfined Aquifer -an aquifer not bound by confining material

Underground Storage Tank- an underground tank storing hazardous substances or petroleum products

Unit of Measure -a predetermined quantity (as of length, time, or heat) adopted as a standard of measurement

Unsaturated Zone -an underground geologic layer in which pores and fractures are filled with a combination of air and water

Volatile Organic Compounds (VOCs) -organic (carbon-based) compounds that evaporate at room temperature

Waste-to-Energy Incinerator -a process unit designed to burn solid, liquid, or gaseous materials under controlled conditions to reduce waste volume and produce energy

Water Table -the upper limit of a geologic layer wholly saturated with water

Water Table Aquifer -an unconfined aquifer in which the water table can rise and fall

Well -a hole sunk into the ground to reach a supply of water